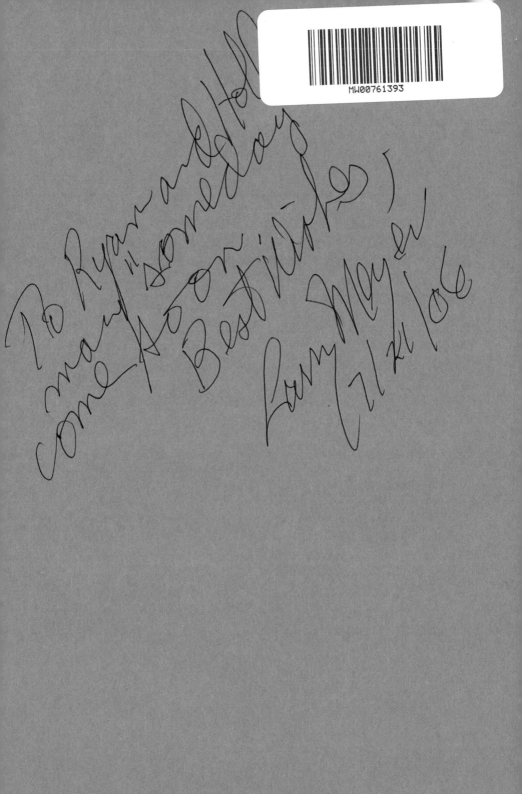

To Ryan and Holly,
may "someday"
come too soon someday.
Best wishes,
Larry Meyer
12/21/06

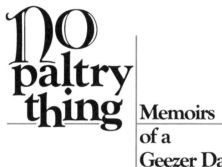

no paltry thing

Memoirs of a Geezer Dad

BOOKS BY THE
SAME AUTHOR

Shadow of a Continent

California Quake

Long Beach:
Fortune's Harbor
(*Co-Authored with
Patricia Kalayjian*)

The Complete Works
of Marcus Uteris

My Summer with Molly:
The Journal of a Second
Generation Father

no paltry thing

Memoirs of a Geezer Dad

by
Larry L. Meyer

"An aged man is but a paltry thing,
A tattered coat upon a stick, unless
Soul clap its hands and sing, and louder sing
For every tatter in its mortal dress...."

W. B. Yeats
Sailing to Byzantium

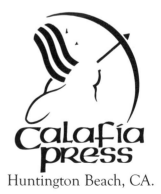

Calafia
press
Huntington Beach, CA.

Library of Congress Cataloging-in-Publication Data

Meyer, Larry L. 1933-
    No paltry thing : memoirs of a geezer dad/Larry L. Meyer.--1st ed.
        p. cm.
    ISBN 0-942273-05-02 (alk. paper)
    1. Middle aged fathers--Psychology. 2. Middle aged fathers--Attitudes
    3. Pregnancy in middle age. 4. Children of older parents. I. Title

    HQ756.M493 2004
    306.874'2'08440973--dc22

                                                      2004050286

For My Family,
Members Living,
Dead, And Yet
To Be

Table of Contents

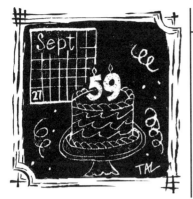

Chapter 1

The Birthday Gift

I COULD BE PREGNANT."

I look into my young wife's face for signs of jest. Did her sometimes-wicked sense of humor encompass telling a budding geezer on the eve of his fifty-ninth birthday that he could be a father for the sixth time? No, she's not that cruel.

"How could you be?"

"Remember when I told you the cap slipped."

My ears may have heard, but the mind must have dismissed it. The odds said not likely. "How late are you?"

"Two days."

"That's not long. You'll probably start tomorrow."

"Probably...but don't you think I should take the test?"

"Sure." Butterflies flutter under my shirt. "Might as well put your mind at ease." My mind could stand some easing, too.

Timarie rushes off to the drugstore to get the test kit. I walk in circles and tell myself the cervical cap didn't slip. The gel didn't fail. Besides, I am so old that my sperm must have dwindled to a short-lived few.

She pours the urine into the little white cup. It vanishes in the small recess. Then she adds the telltale solution.

Memoirs of a Geezer Dad

I feel angina pains. No, not now.

Almost immediately, the liquid takes on a faint pinkish cast.

"Pink isn't the color of positive…is it?"

"Yes, it is."

Maybe I'm not seeing pink. Maybe I'm imagining things. The fluid is just borrowing pink from the bathroom walls…except the walls are a pale lavender. "It's a very light pink, if it is pink," I say, spreading a margin for error.

"Yes, but it looks more pink than white," says the thirty-one-year-old mother of two young girls, a woman who has viewed these home tests with me twice before.

I tingle with sudden satisfaction—precisely the opposite emotion of what I mean to feel. What is going on? Then the surge of euphoria ebbs, and dread returns.

"This test can give false positives, right?"

"I don't know."

"When can you see the doctor?"

"They should be coming back from lunch about now. I'll drive down right now and get the test."

"Today? Right now?"

"Yes. You don't think I could wait a day, do you?"

"No."

I stand by as she gets into the car. "Don't be unhappy," she says.

"I'm not. Just excited and confused."

The mind riots. The better part of 59 years I've tried to manage my emotions, make life obey my wishes, and then this happens, and no one to blame it on…except the cowardly self.

Not two weeks before, I had discussed with my two younger brothers my intent to get a vasectomy. They assured me the surgery was minor. My wife had previously urged me to undergo the procedure. I dithered. Knives, though their cuts be minute, are no friends of mine.

The Birthday Gift

Not two days earlier, I had been romping with my two-year-old Madeleine, thinking bittersweetly how the generative phase of my life should soon, if tardily, pass.

And now this life-disturbing possibility, precipitated by some unplanned late-night frolic following a night at the theater to see *Heartbreak House*. George Bernard Shaw's the cause…the play was the thing. Damn the supporting caffeine that followed!

Why doesn't she call?
She does. "Happy birthday, Big Boy. You're a dad again."
"You're kidding. They can't be sure."
"Dr. Mahato has never seen a false positive."
"When?"
"Due date, September 27."
Pause.
"Well, dear, it's life, and we work with it."
"Yeah."
"We have to stay flexible."
"Uh-huh." *Flexible?*

At my fifty-ninth birthday dinner with my wife and two daughters I make tries at some good-humored bravado over birthday cake, but shafts of depression break through.

"I feel weak I'm in so much shock," Timarie admits after the girls leave the table.

"Multiply that by 27."

"Why are you so glum? It changes *my* life in a big way."

"Yeah, for the better. You're deliriously happy. All your friends are pregnant, and you can't wait to join the crowd again."

Memoirs of a Geezer Dad

"Can't you say anything nice to me?"

"Congratulations earth mother, from this ancient walking sperm bank."

"Will I be able to handle three?"

"You probably will. I won't," I say in a darkening mood.

Two days into the newly changed reality, my wife and I decide to tell our five-year-old daughter, Molly. The little red-headed girl is ecstatic. The prospective sibling's sex seizes her interest. "When are you going to have an intercom to see if it's a boy or girl?" she asks.

"We'll have the ultrasound in three or four months," Timarie corrects the vocabulary error through a suppressed laugh.

"Mom, we need to get set up for this baby."

"Yes, we will," her mother agrees. "And that means we'll all have to help out. You and Madeleine, too."

I'm wondering whether Maddy—another redhead—should be included in this call to cooperation, when Molly turns to me. "Now you're gonna be a father of more children, Dad, probably because they said they're probably sure."

Yeah, kind of…but my delight with Molly's words fades soon enough. Another child…another expense to dilute resources of a man nearing retirement. A child the actuarial tables say I'll see rather little of. And we'll have to re-supply ourselves with A & D Ointment in the industrial tub size.

Name-selection time…. Already? Just a week after the bomb got dropped? Why not? Names given take on more import the closer one gets to death. Perpetuating the memory of departed kin…aunt or uncle, father, mother's maiden name, knowing that soon enough the reasons for the names being given will be forgotten, long before some mindless asteroid snuffs-out human existence…and any would-be escapees from earth will likely not remember that I tried to honor my father.

If it's a girl, which now seems more likely, now that I've had

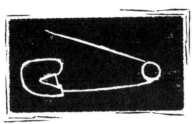

two in a row, following a first-marriage run of three boys (X-sperm swim slower, I've heard, and are more plentiful in older guys). If it's a girl, we winnow the candidates to three: Evelyn, Olivia, or Elise. And a boy? We agree on Franz, after a dear German friend of ours. Besides, its simple one-syllable Teutonicity goes well with my other sons' names: Eric, Kurt, Karl. And then there's the lofty associations with Haydn, Schubert, Liszt, Kafka, not to mention an emperor or two.

Two weeks after the positive test, and I find myself trying not to think about the family's increase by one. Or, God forbid!, two? There's a precedent for that; Kurt and Karl from my first family are twins. The mind flees to easier things…like possibly refinancing the house…a little cash pulled out will come in handy.

"You look unhappy," my wife says. "Let's see a smile."

"Make me smile."

"Pampers."

Memoirs of a Geezer Dad

Mouth relaxes.
"Baby bottles."
Further.
"Two o'clock feeding."
A grin.
"Potty training."
A pained cackle.
"There, you see. Better already."
"If I laugh at any human thing, it is that I may not weep,"
I parrot the poet who shares my birthday.

"Are you really that sad?" my wife asks, concerned and
clearly disappointed with me.

"I'm beyond happy or sad. I just feel...trapped."

A terrible word with which to end a conversation, but
that's it for now as our feelings go their separate ways.

Ultrasound day. The revelation is at hand, and we will
confront it as a family. Some couples don't want to know the
gender; we do. Some like the thrill of waiting until birth; not
me. A crowning and then emerging head is thrill enough.

Timarie is sky-high, Molly is on her patented intelligence
alert, Madeleine is distracted by strange objects in the ultrasound lab, and I am in calm paralysis, my usual defensive pos-
ture these days.

I watch the cheerfully chattering technician jelly Tim's
belly and turn on the machine. As in the two previous preg-
nancies, I have trouble making sense of the light and dark
patches on the screen in this search for the sought object, but
the tech calls out what she's measuring—femurs, kidneys,
brain. "Brain looks good," she says, and—though I wonder
how she could possibly know such a thing—I feel good, as I did

when young and thought my get would lighten the human lot. Now I worry about leaving my own as unsupervised burdens on a society with holes in its pockets.

Molly keeps asking whether the blob under scrutiny is a boy or a girl, while the tech puts her off with "what-would-you-like-it-to-be?" counter questions. The woman glances at me, fishing for a preference. I don't comment, because I'm not sure, and "none-of-the above" is not on the answer sheet, though I had a dream just days before that it was a boy.

Finally, the tech moves the cursor to a small white nib. "There it is—a penis. I thought it was a boy earlier."

Molly strains to see this mysterious property.

"Are you sure?" Timarie asks, incredulous.

"Yes."

"I didn't think you could be sure. A friend told me you can't be sure because sometimes the female genitalia can be enlarged due to hormones in utero and can look like a penis."

"Was the friend a trained technician?" the woman, herself seven months pregnant with a boy, counters.

End of discussion.

A boy! O my prophetic soul! The improbable has become confirmed reality. And how does my weird mind react? I immediately process the in-utero child's sex into the extended Meyer family breakdown of males to females, and note that the three-generation-old 2–1 male-to-female ratio has been restored. All's right with the world. Mathematics can be so reassuring.

Not for long. Will my arthritis allow me to teach Franz to play baseball? Even hit a Tee Ball? Will he survive the trauma of my death? Boys are fragile that way.

Timarie's euphoria buoys me some for the next few weeks. So my sixth child will arrive as I close on my sixtieth year. The die is cast. Family will be the focus of my life as never before, and tending three young children will be my overtime job. Chin up, *mon brave!*

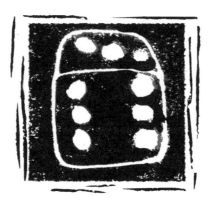

Two months pass, and what is imminent can't be deferred completely. A sign of Tim's nesting is her increased badgering of me to get a long-overdue cholesterol check, which I resist out of plain male obstinacy—and the family fault of avoiding doctors so they can't discover a fatal or threatening dysfunction that only materializes when you seek out their counsel. So I give in to the nagging and go get the expected bad news. Namely, that in spite of an overall healthful diet light on meats, sweets, and dairy products, my cholesterol count remains higher than Babe Ruth's lifetime batting average. A genetic legacy I can't control with any existing remedy. Gloom hinting at doom.

I confront guilt behind my pessimism. Have I done wrong bringing another life into a sinking world? This is not post-adolescent *Weltschmerz*, but a reasoned appraisal of the world I see, overpopulated and undereducated, hungry and angry, with human opportunities clearly shrinking before one's eyes. I can't handle the stress, so I try to banish the whole subject of the baby to the periphery of my consciousness, as though it were a horrendous bill due some months off and not worth my immediate worry.

Doesn't work. The prospect of life as a geezer father goads me to think of changing my whole life plan. The recession of 1992 has hit the State of California hard, and the state university system faces financial crisis. Just this June I learned of Sacramento's plan to pension off senior professors—give them some extra years of retirement credits to depart early so they can be replaced with cheap temps and bottom-of-the-ladder assistant professors lacking tenure. I happen to be one of those senior professors, teaching journalism at California State University Long Beach, working in an environment of plunging morale, and weary of the petty politics that poison the halls of higher learning. Could I retire early? My wife works a decent job. I could stay home with my last child—enjoy what will never be again. But I would have to supplement our income somehow. Back to freelance writing? Back to my years of living dangerously, which kept me on the lip of poverty for five years with my first family? And what about health insurance? What if the baby has—God forbid!—"health problems," that unsettling euphemism for at least 500 natural shocks that flesh is heir to? Can I really risk such a life change when all this is up in the air? There's only a few months' window on the early retirement option, so I'll have to decide soon.

The month of September begins a new semester and ends the baby-on-the-back-burner state of mind. My wife, who has sensed my deep misgivings about becoming a father so late in life, but is optimist enough to believe in my longevity (I ask for assurances of it in writing), confronts me precisely two weeks before her due date. "Hey! What do you think about this

Memoirs of a Geezer Dad

baby? What do you think about our having a little baby boy and son? One of these days I am going to tell you he's coming and you're going to say, 'Great. I can't wait to meet him.' "

Maybe so. But before that, in three days actually, I'm scheduled to see a doctor to discuss the overdue vasectomy. Timarie got the referral, briefly consulted with the doctor, brought back a procedure overview, which she passes along to the great procrastinator. Her thinking? We might as well be celibate—postpartum and post-potent—together, simultaneously.

Sure, it smacks of locking that proverbial barn after the horse has been stolen and all that. But the altering will at least prevent future horses from being at risk. Fertility must have a stop. And I deserve stopping. The most unusual fact of my life is that I have had only eight clear, unobstructed shots at paternity and already have five children—and another on the way—to show for it.

September 16. The real countdown begins. My wife returns from the OB's office and tells me Franz now weighs seven pounds in utero. I'm instantly lifted by the news. He's very safely viable now, and I instinctively warm to the prospect of a new son. I am beginning to wonder what is really under Timarie's bulge—what the boy will look like. Another redhead, as my own long-dead mother was and my two daughters are? Not likely. That would be like hitting the Triple at Santa Anita. More likely blond…as I was and one of my three previous sons was. With no disfigurements to make his life harder than it has to be, I hope.

September 18. This day I consult with the cutter. The doctor is a slender man in his fifties, professionally affable. His mind seems fixed on dutifully addressing my fears of surrendering my fertility and allaying them. I admit the thought has troubled me some on a deep and primitive level. But other concerns step forward.

I interrupt his practiced lecture. I explain that I'm about to have my sixth child, an unplanned child, as I near age 60, and I can handle the trauma of not being a new daddy again. My real worry, I explain with shamed face, is that I am a coward. At least when it comes to being cut. In my whole life I've only had two minor surgeries—tonsils taken out at seven and a triggered thumb repaired at 55. It's the physical pain I fear, the prospect of which deterred me from having a vasectomy the previous December, during a between-the-semesters' window of opportunity just a week or two before a frisky sperm got through all the lets to meet by chance a receptive egg.

The doctor assures me the pain will be minimal. Recovery will be short. Complications are rare. So we set a date in October.

September 22. Unlike the young parent who sees the coming baby as a sign of life and hope, I'm overtaken by a certain morbidity. I'm aware that birth is a prelude to death, with life tucked in between, and for me the chain ends at the grave's edge. If only it were otherwise. If only someone or something would send me a sign that the chain is circular, unbroken, I would hope, too.

September 23. Today I give in to Timarie's continued harassing and haranguing and show up at the doctor's appointment she's scheduled for me. I go with grumbles and my usual fear that he will discover I've only two days to live. When I tell the Doc why I'm there, he grins. "She wants a father for her baby, huh?"

Memoirs of a Geezer Dad

The prescription? With a new statin family drug (the previous have brought crippling side effects) we will try to get my cholesterol count down from 350 to well below 300. (Sure…but a counter wisdom circulates in my mind—why not a quick exit from a heart attack, with all the life insurance premiums paid up?)

September 24. Today my bulging wife Magic Markers my lunch bag with "Father of Franz," as though I need a reminder as I head to a school faculty meeting of what is imminent. I really must psyche myself up to receive my last child warmly. To be sure, my curiosity about who he will be is heating up by the hour.

September 26. This is the anniversary date of the death of my father, gone nine years. Though I ridicule others' belief in signs and superstitions, I have this rare premonition that Franz Lawrence Meyer will be, fittingly, born of this day…bring some consoling symmetry to my life. Am I hunting omens as aging gnaws at my natural skepticism?

Timarie starts feeling her first contractions at about 1 p.m. She packs for the hospital, then tries to nap as the early labor proceeds sluggishly. Time for a leisurely house cleaning, doing the laundry, and packing Molly and Madeleine off for brief a stay with Auntie Lisa. It isn't until 8:55 p.m., with the contractions five minutes apart, that Timarie and I depart for the hospital . But they slip to six as I miss the oft-traveled turnoff to the hospital and have to double back a mile. Stress? Or creeping senility?

Check-in is quick, routine. Timarie is up, cocky. We guess on dilation. Timarie says three; I say two. It's one millimetering toward two.

At 9:15 the fetal monitor is strapped on and we get ready for the event, though the September 26 arrival date no longer seems likely. Then the contractions weaken, stretch out to ten-minute intervals. After an hour of arrested progress, we are sent home sheepish for an anticlimactic day's end of television-news watching and then to bed.

September 27. Tim is panicky at 7:07 a.m. She's spent all night up and down, and now she's up with a vengeance. "Time to go!" No, there is no time for my shower. "Brush your teeth and be done with it!" Should I call the paramedics for help? That would be the coward's way out. "Let's go!" is her stern command.

So at 7:14 we're off, and I think I'm pretty composed under the circumstances, though the traffic lights are not kind. Tim is sucking in her breath, telling me to hurry. My knees feel spongy. Don't tell me I'm going to be one of those local-feature-page fools with firemen delivering the baby roadside as I gawk on! Firemen? Where did they come from? More likely, the critical task would fall to me, and I'm clearly not up for it.

At 7:25 I ease up to the emergency entrance, and at Tim's urging to rush, attendants materialize with a wheelchair.

"Hurry!" Timarie bleats again. Me? The medics? All of us probably, so I hit the brake for the quick unload, then pull the car into a nearby parking slot and rush through the Pre-Admit Entrance after the birthing party. In a heart-thumping trot I catch up with my wife as she is wheeled into a labor and delivery room.

"Who's your doctor?" a first nurse asks as Tim is helped into a bed.

"Dr. Mahato," she says through grinding teeth. They have

the number on file. A second nurse moves into an adjacent closed-off area to make the call.

"You're six," Nurse #1 says to Timarie. She turns to Nurse #2 and announces gravely, "If her water breaks, we have a baby."

Now? What do *I* do? Hold her hand as she groans through another contraction.

"Do you want an epidural?" Nurse #1 asks.

"Absolutely!" Timarie says with fervor, in what seems half-plea, half-instruction.

Another contraction, and mother-to-be and Nurse #1 layer their exclamations. Forget the epidural. The water has broken. Shock time.

"Get the Emergency Room doctor," says Nurse #1 to Nurse #2. God! How long is that going to take?

"Don't push! Don't push!" exhorts Nurse #1.

"I won't!" my wife screams, fighting another contraction.

Shouldn't the nurse be experienced enough to do the delivery? She moves between Tim's legs ready to do that very thing, when the emergency doctor enters. He's young and appears hesitant to me. Nurse #2 jokingly puts words to my fears: "Are you ready?" God almighty! Not some resident radiologist-to-be on Emergency Room duty!

The doctor smiles, bends down, and examines the work ahead of him. Tim pushes once. Out scoots a head. A pause as the doctor works his hands scissors-fashion, then the shoulders emerge, followed by a sudden smooth expelling of tiny limbs. Done. Not 15 minutes in the hospital, after only nine contractions, Franz is arrived.

But I hear no immediate sound, no cry as the doctor works over him. Stillborn?

The mask is put on the lethargic little form to suck out the mucous. "Awaaa," comes the first faint cry.

Hallelujah! He's alive, and I'm alive, and I haven't disgraced myself in this test of my mettle, this unplanned experiment in true natural childbirth!

The doctor cuts and clamps the cord, then hands the swaddled bundle to Tim, and the little guy with the merest suggestion of blond stubble on his pate starts nursing at first asking.

I stand wooden among the happy bustle attending my wife and son, too stunned to really note what is taking place. Then Nurse #2 suddenly hands him to me. "Hey Dude!" are my involuntary words of greeting, invoking that hackneyed noun I've long disliked and criticized my other sons for using. "You're among friends," I say to reassure him. I hold him through the wraps, kiss his head through his cap. Joy fills my chest cavity.

"He looks like you," Nurse #1 says.

How can she tell? "He cries like me," I admit. That brings general laughter.

"His lungs are rattling—I feel it in his back," I announce to the just-arrived Dr. Mahato, who is relieving the emergency room doc.

She checks his pale back and chest with the stethoscope, then reassures me there's nothing amiss.

Wow! This day begun in hectic worry—this clear and sunstruck Sunday—has yielded to a general feeling of exhilaration. Undeadened by any painkillers, wife and son are awake, alive and full of pep.

I inspect Franz Lawrence Meyer more closely. At 8 pounds 9 ounces and 21 inches long with his legs straightened out, this blue-eyed little fellow is bigger than I would have expected. His skull is like mine, with enough errant lumps and knobs to keep a team of phrenologists in learned papers for a decade.

He's obviously also a prompt little guy, dropping in on us on his due date. So he wasn't born a day earlier on my father's death date to honor the man whose first name he

Memoirs of a Geezer Dad

will have for his middle (and honor Timarie's father, whose surname is also Lawrence). But then I had similar hopes for my daughter Madeleine Jeannette, born July 27, a day after my mother's death date, who bears my mother's name for her middle.

Just missed twice. Late a day in both instances—there's a pattern in itself. Comforting to someone who hunts for rhythms, design, closed circles, any sign of order that suggests purpose in his universe. What a day!

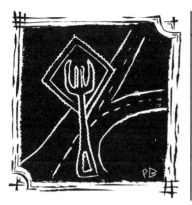

Chapter 2

Forks
in the
Road

THE GENERAL EUPHORIA following a birth quickly yields to the hard work of caring for the newborn—feeding, changing, cleaning, walking on little cat feet through naps, and serving Mom in bed whatever her exhausted body needs to recover. Your own beaten frame has a way of collapsing at about 8:30 p.m., with at least one major disturbance sure to come before the dreaded 2:00 a.m. feeding. Life changes beg to be made.

Yogi Berra said, "When you come to the fork in the road, take it."

Clearly, he had me in mind. Siring a child on the brink of one's sixtieth birthday invites some lifestyle changes and forces some hard choices.

No longer could I put off the decision of what I would do with the rest of my life. Putting extra pressure on me was the fact that I was next in line to become chair of my academic department at CSULB, a "promotion" my wife strongly opposed. The added duties and increased pressure would take me from an already hectic family life made all the more complicated by Franz's arrival. Moreover, my department was not on the university's "preferred list" during the budget crunch, and I already had proved myself a vulnerable novice in the Byzantine world of academic politics. Could I really preserve the department and its budget from powerful administrators looking to cut it down to size? I had real doubts and worries galore.

25

Memoirs of a Geezer Dad

Why not just bail out?, my wife dared to suggest.

Why not indeed! Pull the ripcord and be clear of it all. The State of California was offering a tantalizing incentive to do just that. If I did accept what was being called the "golden handshake" of goodbye (really more a lead parachute painted gold), so that new and cheaper blood could be brought in and abused as part-time instructors and untenured lecturers, I would get at least a couple of additional years of service credit toward my retirement pension. Even more important, I would be able to keep my superior PERSCare health insurance plan to cover myself and my family in the future.

My wife and I sat down at the kitchen table and did the old plusses and minuses balancing act. With the nation in a recession, it would be risky for a family of five to try living on one salary and a monthly pension check much reduced from what the state university had been sending; moreover, Social Security benefits were still five years off. Of course, we would also save on gasoline and eliminate child-care costs, and I could more economically run the household by wise shopping and cooking, avoiding the routine waste of too-tired-to-cook eat-outs with the subsequent "throw-outs" of groceries bought only to gather mold in the vegetable freshener. I could always become a freelance writer again, defined the first time I tried it as a person with a typewriter and a working spouse, now redefined for me as a possessor of a word processor and a young wife blossoming in her editing career. Maybe I could make a go of it this time. Stay home, keep house for my three newest hostages to fortune, and write while I waited for my modest pensions to kick in.

Of course, there were downsides—Little League and Indian Guides again and all the embarrassments I'd cause Franz as a do-nothing, creaky, tag-along Dad...and that only as long as my knees held out. Add those middle-of-the-night rushes to the hospital with fears—unfounded, so far—that a child's limb or lungs hung in the balance.

On the other hand, the California ethos encourages one to change his life at the drop of a name—"re-invent oneself," as the pop-psyche cant goes. So why not become a mature stay-at-home caregiver? No less than T. S. Eliot had said old men ought to be explorers.

In the end, viscera triumphed over the forebrain. I would go back to basics. Make the most of my sixth and last chance at fatherhood. Squeeze the life out of each day I had left living, close to the hearth in loving closeness with my family, my own. All that sort of mush and gush.

My colleagues in the journalism department showed some surprise when I announced at the first faculty meeting after Franz's birth that I would be retiring early. But it was already tempered with a general puzzlement that I, a seemingly reasonable man who professed a belief in choice, would opt to even have a child at my age. This was California, after all—home base of freedom and choice. Probably had the kid at the wife's insistence, they must have reasoned. Maybe because her Catholicism didn't allow abortion.

They missed the point. Choice also meant you could choose, as my wife and I did, to have the child. Strangely, neither she nor I ever even mentioned the abortion option through the strained months from conception to birth. Was it early religious training? A factor, perhaps, but with Timarie all babies are wonders made for her to mother; she could be counted on to love what hap had sent.

For me, was it in deference to my wife's wishes and an unwillingness to risk domestic harmony by even bringing the idea up? No, it went much deeper than her feelings or the teachings of an organized religion. Thanatophobia has hounded me since I was capable of self-reflective thought. I just couldn't allow to be erased a life in which I had half a genetic stake; I couldn't assent to scrape from a uterine wall some mute inglorious Milton who might fill my yearnings for even a marginal immortality. I fear death and hate oblivion too much for that.

There remained another fork to take, another decision on which to follow through: the life-altering cut with its date certain. And so on an October day of broken tropic skies and unseasonable rain showers, the deed got done. No one would ever upstage my Franz.

Not much to the outpatient procedure, really. Uncomfortable needle-pricking of the scrotum, snipping, sewing up (a little sensitivity there). After ten minutes of calculated not-watching, I satisfied my curiosity with a few quick glances. I was sent home for a few days' rest and relaxation as an altered man. In the car I butchered to myself Chief Joseph's eloquence: "From this day forward, I shall breed no more forever." About time, too. On the other hand, I was glad I had waited as long as I had.

My wife sensed my thoughts as she drove me home and asked a question she had asked weeks earlier, to which I had given a weak, unsatisfactory reply in the affirmative.

"Are you glad we have the baby?"

"Yes, I am." I assured her.

"You know, if we had lost Franz, I would have had to have another child." Strong and unsettling words that could now be ignored.

Forks in the Road

But we hadn't lost him. So now he would have to be fine. What was done couldn't be reversed without more complicated, expensive, and painful surgery, and even then there would be no guarantees, my cutter had said.

Someday, long after I'm gone, Timarie will have to tell Franz that he owes his very existence to his father's unmanly fear of minor surgery and the lively wit of George Bernard Shaw.

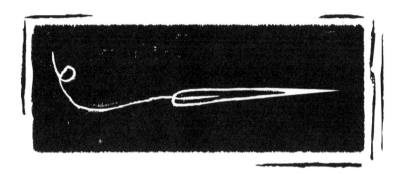

On January 22, 1993, I spent my sixtieth birthday cleaning out my office, with its 15 years of accumulated clutter—mostly old final exams and term papers from a broad range of courses. Down from the walls came the framed honors and degrees. Down came the posters bearing advice from A. J. Liebling and Albert Camus, two of my century's worthiest journalists. And down came the cartoons by Charles Schulz and Gary Larson and Tom Wilson posted for my amusement by students. I would miss them most…America's young men and women and the classroom give-and-take they provided that kept the mind sharp and open. What a fine and reassuring adventure it had been to teach writing, editing, ethics and literature to them. Media hand-wringing to the contrary, the nation's future was in good hands, and the future would be better than the past. At least that was the faith I was taking away from the university.

Memoirs of a Geezer Dad

Surfacing through this roil of wistful thinking was a line from writer Gene Fowler. He advised his son that he live life with the intensity of children and poets and jaguars. I had lived so in the past. But now I was turning toward home to help my own brood and blood—ages six, three and four months. Was I up to it again? More to the point, could I succeed as a geezer father on the home front, serving as both homemaker and nanny? When I turned in my office key, I noticed a slight trembling of the hand.

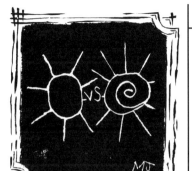

Chapter 3

A
house husband
Again

I BROUGHT HIGH HOPES for new insights to my second round of parenting. But the initial months in my second tour of duty as a paterfamilias seemed little changed. Instead of a station wagon I now drove a minivan—amply supplied with built-in car seats—on my endless daily rounds to and from school, various markets, ballet lessons, gymnastics lessons, half-days spent in doctors' waiting rooms, ensuing trips to the pharmacy for a different antibiotic that might work this time. All done, of course, in the company of tiny tots clamoring for juice, a toy, a change, or just clamoring for the pure hell of it—particularly during the children's hour, when it was best to be off the street. I might as well have been barefoot, pregnant, and housebound than a jitney driver again. My only consolation was that I plied the surface streets during off-hours rather than freeways during the rush-turned-crush.

My new life was begun with the best of professional intentions. Uniquely positioned as an aged parent of little ones, I meant to keep a journal—episodic and sporadic as it would likely be—of what it was like to be a geezer father. It was not just an idle caprice. Yes, I had a book in mind. As the author of six previous books (admittedly, only one on the subject of parenting), I could stay healthy in my craft while passing along to the reckless few considering a similar life-change the fruits of my experiences, which—who knew—might include major revelations, or just some hard-won advice on how to make fathering a bit easier. No surprise that I had a lengthy tome in mind; a short one would

Memoirs of a Geezer Dad

certify my early demise and my second family left fatherless at a tender age.

Such morbid words suggest a second reason—a surmounting reason—for my keeping the journal. It would help my children flesh out memories of their father and the lives we spent together as a not-quite-traditional family…let them know a little of who I was, how I felt about them, leave a record of the daily nitty-gritty of the lives we shared…if only briefly.

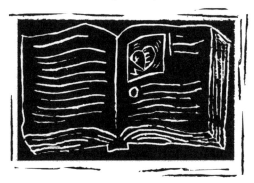

Keeping up with the journal proved difficult. First, there were the constant demands of the three kids and cooking and keeping house. Second, and the telling one, was that I had aged and simply lacked the physical stamina I had raising my first family. It came down to entropy. Energy loss, plain and simple, erodes whatever advances you've made through mental maturation or parenting experience, resulting in a reduction in work output. The clipper snips on the backyard bougainvillea are less frequent and less forceful, and the time to trim the tree—once a mere half-hour—now grows into 50 minutes; the sweat and frustration is not lost upon you. It is so common-place, so predictable, and yet it comes as a shock to witness your own body breaking down, steadily if not rapidly, and it adversely affects you in many ways, ten of which I've taken the trouble to list here:

A houseħusband Again

1. Aging takes the oil out of your joints and leaves ground glass in its place.

2. Aging makes one a major phlegm factory working the full three shifts.

3. Aging crabs your handwriting, which becomes increasingly erratic and you recognize as belonging to an old person.

4. Aging splatters modest leg veins into showy purple spider webs and raises random lumps from limbs that once had fetching curves to them.

5. Aging increases the number of doctor, dental, and lab appointments you must meet to keep the deteriorating corpus from coming completely apart all at once.

6. Aging removes that aggressive set of mind that once served you well in the witty give-and-take of cocktail parties, so that now you always come up with your best "give" two hours after the party is over.

7. Aging makes you forgetful enough to leave your fly open when you no longer have a reason to advertise.

8. Aging sculpts what teeth you have left into a craggy sierra that traps most food particles attempting to pass through and makes dental floss a necessary pocket pal to your wallet.

9. Aging cakes dried snot inside your nostrils, setting up such a god-awful itch that you've got to pick and scrape no matter that the Queen of England is staring straight at you across your dinner salads.

10. Aging flushes from covert body parts rancid juices that stain your clothing and remind you of your last visit to a convalescent home.

Memoirs of a Geezer Dad

There are other effects of a less delicate nature that need not be gone into here.

The best barometer of my mounting physical limitations was the game of horsy. In my stallion's prime I could pack three little boys on my back at once and do the length of the hall in no time flat. First daughter Molly I could carry with some painful huffing and puffing. Half a featherweight Madeleine I could support for a sixth of a furlong on my rickety knees. But when Franz—a young lummox in the making—saddled up, my knees turned to needles, and this graying gelding was ready to be turned out to pasture, with no prospects of further stud service.

Accompanying the physical changes in an aged father are lifestyle changes as well. The person you were is not the person you've become. Ditto for your expectations. Since Stockholm still hasn't called, you need waste no more time polishing your Nobel Prize acceptance speech. Sure, it's a humbling experience to realize you are no Prince Hamlet, nor were meant to be. But it also takes a lot of pressure off. The first time around one's "life work" (also known as career or survival plan) demanded almost all your thoughts and energies. The second you think less and less of yourself and more and more of what your issue might do, and how you can help them. One reason must be that my own life really doesn't require the close attention it once did. I'm not going anywhere I haven't been.

I've discovered other changes. During my first round of parenting I would rise early to get to the typewriter and busy myself with those novels and histories before the din of sibling wars and miscellaneous morning grouchiness broke the silence. Now I rise, still early, to savor the morning calm and silence while I sip coffee and read the sports page. Things that used to absorb me—a good murder mystery, handicapping thoroughbreds—bore me quickly now. What's more likely to engage me is a news item about a cancer-causing gene being discovered in some university lab or an orbiting telescope's confirmation of planets circling other stars in our galaxy.

There are positively positive surprises as well. My fear that I would lack interest in children as children, be too crotchety to pay them much mind, proved false. I find that re-entering the world of a child is not half-bad, as long as I spend quality time with Ernie and Bert and Kermit and SpongeBob and avoid Alvin the chipmunk and the adenoidal whine of Rugrats that seems to penetrate double walls and sets my teeth to grinding.

To the enduring genius of Jim Henson, add the joy of rereading Dr. Seuss to another round of attentive kids, though I advise sticking to *Green Eggs and Ham* and *The Cat in the Hat* and skipping *You're Only Old Once!*

Another benefit, it turns out, the geezer father finds himself more in touch with holidays, anniversaries, inaugurations and like rites that dignify life's commonplace events. Such days seem longer, are made more meaningful.

I even found a bonus in the onerous daily demands of keeping house and raising kids; they kept me so busy and harried that I didn't have time to brood over past failures and just generally feel sorry for myself. Rooting for longevity, I might add that some anecdotal evidence suggests senior folks in loving families live longer than those in adult orphanages.

Of course, these are only first impressions that I hope to build on. I do know that I'm more generous to my children this time around. Why? Because I have the time. I can do what I observe in most grandparents…giving in little ways, truly concerned with easing and guiding the lives of loved ones who live after me. It's so wonderful being home and able to go to your child's noon kindergarten "graduation" and watch the red-headed girl—already winner of the perfect attendance award—beam for the class picture, wearing her soul on her fresh face. Oh, the pure and simple misty-eyed joy of it all!

Memoirs of a Geezer Dad

Finally, I should mention a difference in parenting this time that has nothing to do with aging or changing mores. This time I have daughters, and girls really are different from boys. Moreover, as was soon evident to me, there can be great differences in sisters three years apart who share red hair and Celtic skin and the same parents. Luckily, Franz was a good baby, which in parent speak means he slept a lot and therefore cried less. I had just put him down one afternoon for his nap when the noisy backyard battle began. Molly was tearfully berating her younger sister with unaccustomed force. "You cheater!—I hate you!"

Knowing the wisdom of letting sleeping babies lie, undisturbed, I hurried out to silence the combatants and make peace if I could.

"What is this all about?" I demanded in a hushed but authoritative voice.

"Madeleine is a cheater, and she lies!" Molly roared through real tears.

"Shush! You'll wake Franz." I looked down at three-year-old Madeleine; she looked both sheepish and triumphant.

"What happened, Molly?"

Punctuated with further denunciations of her sister's perfidy, she explained. Ever the competitor, Molly had organized an art contest between herself and the next-door neighbor girl Laura, attended by Laura's cousin, Katie. Perhaps with misplaced confidence, Molly had appointed Madeleine judge of this juried show. And little Madeleine had chosen the foreigner's work, with the foreigner's cousin Katie's assent.

"She likes Laura better than her own sister!" Molly said, incredulously. Just recounting the treachery threw her into another red rage, which sent the victorious artist and her loyal cousin home in a quiet rush.

"Madeleine is entitled to her own opinion," I said. I tried

to explain that one could never really argue matters of taste anyway. "And besides, critics are rarely fair," I added, with a smile for myself.

Making light of the treason made Molly even angrier. I could read the face. Was even her Dad to turn on her?

"You come and look," she challenged. "You'll see that she lies!"

Okay, I agreed to double as art critic and Solomon. Yes, I would look at the artwork and try to be impartial. Perhaps it was Madeleine's judgment and reputation that were problematical.

Following the end of Molly's finger, I inspected the cinder-block wall; two sets of chalk drawings appeared to be depictions of the sun. Clearly, the one on the right, with its well-defined four-part inner core of yellow, gold, purple, and pink was both more sophisticated and a better likeness.

"This one is better." I chose right, and Molly smiled through her vindication.

"Now look at the rainbows."

I did as bade. One was colorfully and clearly what it meant to be. The other showed an uncertain wander of smudged lines suddenly bent over double, as if suffering from stomach cramps. I chose the colorfully traditional one. Right again.

I looked at Madeleine to see what effect my in-the-blind counter judgment had on her. Outside of the sulk that greeted my first entry into the fray as peacemaker, she revealed nothing. I quit the scene as the ongoing bickering died down slowly over the balance of the afternoon and evening.

The next day I began to worry. What if the incident became one of those never-to-be-forgotten and unresolved wrongs of childhood ("I'll never forget that day I caught you stealing a half-dollar from my drawer!") that separate siblings later in life? I decided to check back with the pair and smooth things out, if I could.

First I approached Madeleine in private. "Did you really like Laura's drawings better than Molly's?"

"I liked Molly's best," she confessed.

"Why?"

"Because they were prettier."

"Then why did you choose Laura's? Because you didn't want to hurt her feelings?"

"No." She had turned down my convenient explanation that she was behaving as any proper hostess would.

"Then why?" For reasons unknown to me, her lips remained sealed, and no further interrogation got me so much as a word.

So I went to Molly. "Are you still mad at Madeleine for choosing Laura's art over yours?"

"No," she said to the accompaniment of a don't-be-silly, it's-water-under-the-bridge smile.

"Why do you think she chose Laura's over yours?" (I had already decided that the little one was exacting some overdue vengeance on a bossy big sister.)

"Because she likes Laura and wants to be her friend" was her matter-of-fact answer. A typical logical explanation from a normally logical young lady.

It was time for me to level. "Honey, I just wanted you to know that I thought your sun was *much* better than Laura's."

Her look turned to one of sudden impatience. "It wasn't a sun, Dad. At first it started to be the sun. But then I made it God—my idea of God."

It was time for me to do the dishes. Two days later, as I hosed off the wall and gave my own Nobel Prize to the inventor of erasable chalk, I took a last long look at God the sun. Maybe art couldn't hold my Molly. Theology probably beckoned. As for Madeleine, she had the making of a splendid critic.

A House Husband Again

That was only a tepid introduction to female sibling rivalry. Having had only boys the first time and witnessing on a daily basis competitions that often got downright physical, I had assumed girls were somehow different. They are, but only in the way the rivalries play out, which makes a strong case for nature over nurture.

I continued to do my best handling their dueling, jumping from corner to corner, hearing complaint and counter-complaint, a Solomon in BarbieLand.

Molly: "When we play pretend, Madeleine always wants to be the prettiest girl. Even if there is only one girl, she makes me be the boy. When Laura comes, Maddy insists on being the teacher, and when we get called on for her questions, even if Laura is wrong and I am right, she tells Laura she is right. And she refuses to let it be my birthday."

Sol: "Maybe she's just being hospitable. I'm sure she loves you more."

Madeleine: "Molly is bossy. She always tries to tell me what to do."

Sol: "She is your older sister. I think she's just trying to help you out."

Molly: "When we play 'Birds of America,' we look for birds we would want to be, and you can only be one bird. Madeleine decided to be the swan; I decided to be the eagle. She thought the eagle was ugly. She always insists on being the swan, unless I say we can't be water birds, then she chooses to be an American egret."

Sol: "It's great that you both have such vivid imaginations—a sign of creativity. I like to think of you as birds of a feather—ha-ha—but if she insists on being the egret, then I think you have every right to be the swan."

Madeleine: "Molly is stuck-up. She thinks she is so smart, and she's not."

Memoirs of a Geezer Dad

Sol: "But she is, and she has the grades to prove it. You're smart, too, Maddy, and you can show it by studying hard."

Molly: "Madeleine always makes her dresses not much of a match and makes herself look terrible. From the Barbie's help, she learned to brush and put in ponytails, though she makes them look quite raggedy. The colors do not match well, and she looks like a nerd, though she thinks she looks beautiful."

Sol: "I think your sister has a sense of style and likes to show her individuality in the imaginative way she dresses."

Madeleine: "Molly is ugly. She's got freckles all over her."

Sol: "Molly is not ugly. She's pretty. Most redheads have freckles, and I notice you have some, too, on your nose and on your cheekbones. You're both gorgeous."

Molly: "Madeleine is sneaking Mom's lipstick. And her nail polish. When I caught her, she started saying it was her own. She thinks she's very pretty and I don't think there's a cure for it. She also likes Mom's bra, and she takes my tops and stuffs toilet paper in them and lets the straps show."

Sol: "Really? Mom should be told about that."

It was my cue to leave the minefield for the La-Z-Boy and take in a ball game. Mrs. Solomon could take over the case when she got home from work.

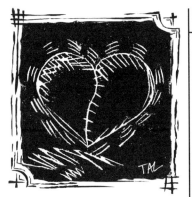

heartaches

O N January 1, 1990, father to a three-year-old daughter and a six-month-old daughter, I belatedly acted on that oft-uttered saw that if I knew I was going to live so long I would have taken better care of myself. I quit drinking. Cold turkey. Sipped a last Kirin beer while watching the Rose Bowl Game and swore off Bombay gin and Martell cognac and all the other delicious poisons I'd sampled amply for 40 years. Ten years before that I had given up smoking cigarettes, after 27-years' pack-a-day addiction to the evil weed. Also done cold turkey.

It's absolutely amazing what the fear of death can accomplish!

At the risk of being redundant, geezer fathers know mortality is their mortal enemy. Offsetting that modest collective virtue, I personally come from a long line of males who do not go to doctors for the very simple and rational reason that you don't go shopping for bad news. (Back in my salad days, when I would return home from an infrequent medical checkup with a no-cancer lung picture and a decent kidney scan, I celebrated by lighting up a Herbert Tareyton and pouring myself a double Bombay on the rocks to toast my continued luck and good health.)

The unexpected arrival of Franz gave me new incentives to stick around, further impetus to mend my ways. I first tried to develop my own preventive-care regimen. I watched what I

41

ate. Exercised almost daily. Learned *T'ai chi chih* to reduce stress. Nevertheless, the need to modestly add to my life insurance, with the requisite exams, not to mention the general physical deterioration associated with aging, forced me to visit doctors more often. Sure enough, they found the fly in my ointment. My cholesterol—the LDL bad kind—and trigly cerides were at astronomical levels. How could that be? There was the exercise. Moreover, being lactose-intolerant, I didn't drink milk, was allergic to cheese and ice-cream and most deserts worth eating. In truth, I favored fruits, vegetables, lean meats and whole grains in my diet. Why the high score? Turns out, my elevated cholesterol was a genetic condition, a curse I shared with my siblings. What should I do?

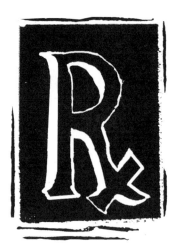

I tried changing GPs. But the high counts followed me, and the lipid-lowering drugs Lopid and Pravachol prescribed savaged me with severe muscle pain and other immobilizing symptoms. I went to the hospital once to check my gall bladder; Krohn's disease was also a suspect. Tests for both proved negative, thankfully.

Heartaches

Then came the summer of 1995. I found that after a half-mile of brisk walking a strange contraction under my breastbone would stop me and sit me down, gasping for air. Pollens...had to be. Or the smog of August clogging my bronchial tree...though my corner of Southern California is among the most smog-free.

The following month I visited my brothers and sister on the high desert for a family reunion and immediately found myself dizzy and short of breath. The paramedics were called and came to examine me. My heart—always reliable in the past—checked out. But my sister, a nurse, strongly advised that I get myself to a cardiologist. I vacillated, dragged my reluctant feet, until I could not handle the chronic anxiety any longer.

On the day after a cheerless worry-filled Christmas and a month before my sixty-third birthday, I went to a cardiologist for a stress test. The zigzag had an extra zag. Something was amiss. Was I experiencing pain in my neck and jaw? Well, yes, now that you mention it, I was. More tests were ordered for the following week.

I was stunned. Hadn't I had cleaned up my act? Where was the fairness? As a practicing existentialist, I knew, of course, there wasn't any. So the week and a half between my warning treadmill and the first intrusive diagnostic probe was a gray sludgy hell of attempting to put the whole thing out of my mind. Words I had only half-understood—angiogram, cardiolite, Thalium—suddenly were words dividing life from death. My life, my death. So I went home and made my will. And congratulated myself on keeping current on all my life insurance premiums, even while worrying that the benefits were not nearly enough to provide for my survivors.

On January 10, 1996 I took an angiogram on an outpatient basis. The good news was that my heart seemed fine. The bad news was that my coronary arteries were 55% to 85% clogged—

too much for angioplasty. Bypass surgery—which had "low morbidity rates" (shouldn't the word be "mortality"?), according to my cardiologist—was the best if not the only course of action. Did I want to take a week or so to think about it? No, that would be a hell of hells, my wife and I agreed. Better to go right to it.

I didn't even go home, but straight to the hospital for a sedated sleep that could conceivably be my last slumber. "Low morbidity" kept circulating through my mind like a reassuring mantra.

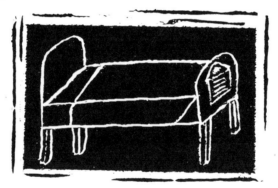

Early the next morning, I received my anesthetic as I was wheeled down the hospital hall toward surgery and my "cabbage"– or Cardio Arterial Bypass Graft. Fear made its appearance on cue. What if I died? A painless death to be sure. But what would happen to my wife? My young daughters? What about my three-year-old son? The questions filtered through the semi-stupor that was my last defense against terror. "Low morbidity" were my last words before the anesthetic took sudden effect.

No morbidity was the outcome. As could have been predicted from being attended by a superior surgeon in a top hospital with the best health insurance coverage the State of California offers—reminders all I was among the nation's blessed, a survivor in that peculiarly American process of natural selection, where those who have good health insurance and good doctors live long and the rest (many living long with chronic ailments that have never been treated) die sooner.

I mended quickly. Through faithful practice of a sound exercise regimen and adherence to a calorie-reduced diet, I became fit enough to not only attend but to dance in joy and thanks at my twenty-nine-year-old son Karl's wedding in May of 1996 and at his twin brother Kurt's wedding in October of the same year.

But the culprit remained, that bad and high cholesterol. With a warning that I should not expect any warm bedside manner, I was referred to a university research specialist in lipids who put me on a parade of statin drugs I hadn't already taken—Lescol, Mevacor, Novocor, Zocor and Lipitor. In a matter of weeks each in turn inflicted severe muscle pain and partial paralysis of my lower body, with nausea an additional side effect. As a last resort the specialist put me on a non-statin drug, Cholestid, which in two months time doubled my cholesterol and rendered me virtually inert.

The specialist was surprised and briefly entertained the idea of doing a paper on me—this rare creature who had bad reactions to all cholesterol-lowering drugs known to medical science—but then discarded it. Better things to do with his time, I guess. He told me he didn't have anything else to suggest. Perhaps I should keep abreast of lipid research and see what other drugs—non-statin variety—might come along in the future.

Might. Might not. I felt wronged, depressed, confirmed in my worst fears of being an old man who gambled on another family and would likely leave his children young and exposed to difficult lives. So my time was borrowed.... But then wasn't everyone's?

Memoirs of a Geezer Dad

I resolved then and since have striven to make the most of what time I have left, loving my wife and raising my kids and counting my blessings every day. Among those blessings, counted early, was validation of my decision to retire from teaching at the university. Had I decided to stay on in academia as head of a besieged department, I sincerely believe I would have died suddenly in the Chair's swivel chair of a busted pump while on the phone with some scheming dean.

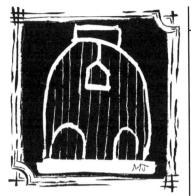

Chapter 5

The Last Menagerie

W̲HEN MY DOG Prunella died in my arms at the pet hospital, I vowed even as the vet withdrew the needle that mercifully ended her losing battle with throat cancer that I would never go through such hell again. If I'd thought a moment, I would have realized that consolation was grounded in unreality. At the time, I was already a second-generation father with a month-old daughter…and with two children to be born three and six years later.

Most families mature in the comforting company of animals—a parade of pets that fill out their days and mark rites of passage. Besides the therapeutic effects of creature companions on lonely adults in need of love, animals introduce children to the wonders of the natural world, teach them respect for life and the inevitability of death.

For me the second parade started modestly enough. My wife wanted a canary for Molly, another presence in our home to brighten our lives with song. Why not?

I got used to the Flutterball, as Molly named the lemon-yellow creature for its nervous antics in its cage. With my wife feeding and watering him and cleaning his cage and covering it at night, he demanded little from me. Moreover, he had a fine voice, reliably cued by the music of Beethoven, which would send him into enchantingly long trills of surpassing beauty. (Good taste, that bird.)

As the years passed and Madeleine and Franz joined the

Memoirs of a Geezer Dad

family, there rose a mounting clamor for more creatures wise and wonderful. Molly complained that all her friends had "real" pets—cats, dogs, turtles, and even pigs. All she had was a canary, who had grown too old even to sing.

True, but I pointed out to Molly that the family wasn't ready to accept the heavy responsibility of caring for a dog, and her father was allergic to cats. No sooner had I made my stand (the last, as it turned out) when fate intervened on Molly's behalf.

A few mornings later, as I drove Molly to school, an odd noise—something akin to a baby's cry—rose from the backseat of the van.

"What is that?" asked Molly.

"I have no idea," I said, leaning forward over the steering column. "Is this one your pranks?" I challenged, suspecting a wind-up doll had been tripped into action.

"Of course not!" Molly protested. "Maybe it's a dying possum," she guessed after listening a little while longer to the morose appeals.

My neck stiffened, my skin crawled with galvanic bumps as I crouched farther forward. Then I pulled over to the curb and stopped the vehicle, got out and pulled open the sliding side door. Out hurtled an enraged cat that brushed my face and hightailed it over a neighbor's fence with cries of defiance.

"Whoa!" gasped Molly.

"Good riddance!" I muttered. I then lectured my daughter about how foolish it was to leave car windows open over night.

The next day the stowaway cat showed up again, this time in our backyard. It was a female tabby of middling size, apparently abandoned by a former owner who had gone to the expense of declawing her front and back. It wouldn't leave, so Molly and her mother started secretly feeding it odds and ends, despite my objections. In a few days a cardboard box was set out in the patio as a bunk for her nocturnal use. Surly and self-

absorbed, she lurked around the yard by day, eyeing me hostile-
ly. I sized her up right away as a typical cat who would allow us
to care for and pamper her for absolutely nothing in
return...save an occasional hiss.

But at least she was not allowed inside, for Dad was allergic
to cats.

After Clea (as Molly named her, short for Cleopatra, which
Molly mispronounced clea-patra) knocked over our trashcans
looking for food, Mom put her foot down. She sent me out to
buy some fancy canned cat dinners, and the beast was as good
as ours...or theirs.

"Don't you just love her?!" Molly asked me.

"She has all the personality of a wet boot," I responded acid-
ly. At least she was an outside cat.

Alas, not for long. As the weather cooled, with increasing
frequency Clea turned up inside in her sleeping box. Enough!

I called a family meeting, and after reprising the lecture
about the itching and sneezing cat dander caused me, I said
with full measure of patriarchal authority, allowing no one any
wiggle room, "Either the cat goes, or I go!"

They must have written it off as bluster. Or else they made
a choice so cruel they couldn't even share it with me. In any
case, without any discussion, Clea soon became a housecat
whenever she wanted our company, which fortunately wasn't as
often as my doting children wished. She preferred roaming the
neighborhood at night, ruling its walls and facing down any
tom that dared cross her path.

I admit I briefly entertained the idea of telling the family I
was renting an apartment, and that I would visit them week-
ends, providing the cat was put out. But I so often saw them
stroking and snuggling the frigid Clea that I couldn't deny their
need to care for and love animals. How else would they learn
the meaning of compassion and touch those dim visceral mem-

Memoirs of a Geezer Dad

ories of a time when humans lived at par with all creatures great and small?

The kids, for their parts, thought that because I hadn't collapsed and died in a sneezing, wealed heap, they had cured me of my allergies—a feat Molly celebrated later in a writing class essay in which I was described as "adaptive."

Apparently emboldened by their healing powers, and against my protestations that one cat was enough, my wife and kids conspired to accept—free, without charge!—a just-weaned kitten from the family next door, another tabby that they christened Marie. Marie must have thought she was a dog. From the start she returned all their strokes and kisses in kind. No surprise then that all the one-way affection previously lavished on Clea was now directed to the diminutive Marie, who made four instant adoring friends. Even my dog-favoring heart was won over in a matter of days by this tiny, noisy extrovert with the cute face.

Marie seemed to know she had moved into first in the hearts of her family. A marvel it was to see the feisty little ball of gray fur in constant pursuit of Clea, who seemed totally discombobulated by the kitten's sass. Meowing fiercely and with claws out, Marie would chase the hulking bully away from their common food dish and just generally torment her much larger roomie.

Maybe the talons were the difference. Maybe Marie was just too constant and energetic a nag. In either case, I was happy to see the family transferring its affections from the grouchy old taker to the playful young giver.

But was justice being done? Okay, so you say what's a canary without a cat. But how do you justify two cats?

Nature, in her wondrous ways, heard my legitimate complaint. Within a few weeks of Marie's coming, Clea began to roam from view. At two months she disappeared completely.

The Last Menagerie

We spent a few agitated days combing the neighborhood for her. In vain. Although we feared the worst, grief remained suspended—and perhaps even lessened—by uncertainty.

Ten days passed before the neighbor lady from two doors down knocked on the door bearing bad news. She had found our missing Clea's body under a front-yard stand of bushes.

What had happened? We didn't know. From what my wife could see of the stiffened corpse, she had not been stuck by a car, as we had feared; her body was intact. More likely it was from natural causes...or some neighbor's poison for snails or rodents...if that's natural. Then again, Clea was a night-fighting wanderer, and there were other possibilities.

My grief was muted, of the sympathetic kind—directed toward my children who would take it hard. My wife and I debated telling them of the grisly discovery. I was for not telling them; let the chance of her leaving us for a better place remain a lingering possibility, and the certainty of death consigned to the future's shadows.

Timarie disagreed. She didn't want the kids to think the cat left us because she preferred another home. More importantly, and wisely I guess, she thought the children should be exposed to life's ultimate reality, the mortality of all living things. (The unspoken subtext, of course, was that Clea's death would prepare them for others' to come...most likely mine, if the law of averages play out.)

How could I argue against such rational thinking? We did agree, however, not to have the kids view the remains, which were attended by the unpleasant aroma of decomposition. Let them remember her in her full, self-assured stalking best, terrorizing other neighborhood felines out of sheer meanness—the "boss cat" of the neighborhood, as Molly dubbed the de-clawed brawler.

My wife phoned Animal Regulation. They sent a man to

remove the body. Then my wife gently broke the news to the kids, who took it rather well, over all. Just a few tears and regrets and prayers and the charming Marie to fill the void.

I was relieved that a negative had been turned into a positive. A life lesson had been learned by all. And at relatively little cost ($40 to Animal Regulation for picking up Clea's carcass), according to this hard-hearted, penny-pinching, dog-lover's reckoning. The cost seemed even less when you figured in that her replacement, Marie, as the kids insist, does have a nice smile.

That lesson? What lives must die, as we were to learn again soon, but with a warning this time.

"I feel sorry for Flutterball," lamented my five-year-old Franz one morning. "Nobody pays attention to him."

He was mostly right. Our nine-year-old, blind-in-one-eye canary, who shed feathers the way Type A human males lose hair and had not sung for over a year, had been neglected by his young keepers, sometimes going a whole day without having his night shroud lifted from his cage.

"Molly pays attention to him sometimes," my son said aloud, as if to soften the hurt of his guilt.

"Yes," I agreed.

"I looked at him a long time once," he followed, apparently still salving his conscience.

"You should do it more often…and soon," I prodded.

My wife had already warned me and the kids that Flutterball would die soon. And she would know. Born to run a bird hospice, she had doctored him through his many physical ailments, diagnosing his blindness early, removing from his slight body ingrown quills with her deft surgical hand, applying salve to his dry feet—even after he had ceased to trill his lovely repertoire because testosterone levels dipped to where unanswered courting songs had nothing behind them. Needless to say, I felt a certain kinship-through-age with the moribund bird.

The morning after Franz's guilt trip, Flutterball died.

My wife, his attentive nurse to the end, found him a disheveled pile of feathers and blood (from intestinal bleeding, it appeared) at the bottom of his cage at breakfast time. Her grief was immediate and teary and spread in only slightly less emotional form among the children as they prepared for school.

Once the kids were off to class, Timarie's mourning went into high shriek. Had she been responsible in any way, she kept asking me. "No, you kept him alive beyond his time," went my reassurances. To no avail. Sobbing went into snuffling. She was taking me down with her.

Then I remembered the lesson of the cats—Clea and Marie. "Why don't you go out and buy another canary—right now," I suggested from a moment of insight.

"Should I?"

"Yes, right now. Bring life in to replace life."

Surprisingly, off she went, to return two hours later without tears and with a new birdcage and a new bird for it—a frisky red canary.

"He was the most lively one the bird farm had," she said. "What shall we name him?"

"How about Carmine?"

"Carmine…I like that. Carmine Flutterheart. Yes, that will be his name." She immediately went into a two-hour flurry of "nesting" in which a corner of living room was antiseptically cleaned, and fresh food and new bird furniture were readied for the new tenant. Marie, already an ace with three proven back-yard bird-kills, observed it all from the hall with special interest.

The kids' return from school was the start of an upbeat two hours as they got to know the newest member of the family. We agreed he was a robust fellow, leaning toward the orange from the red. I lit a log in the fireplace. Marie watched from half-a-room away.

"The man at the bird farm said he would start singing within a month," Timarie said. "If he doesn't, we can bring him back and get another."

At that moment Marie made a lunge for the cage that quarter-turned it and elicited cries of alarm around. Immediate "bad-cat" scolds sent her scurrying; then we reminded one another that she was only doing what nature bade her. Still, if we were to find out whether Carmine would live to make his singing debut, steps would have to be taken. Coins were put in a Coke can to make a rattle that would frighten Marie off. We would all have to be on the qui vive and prepared to shake the can.

The next afternoon, as I was alone reading in the living room, a loud and lilting vibrato trill filled the room. "He's singing!" I yelled to my wife, who was working at the other end of the house. He stopped before she arrived. But a half-hour later, when she returned from school with the kids, Carmine performed an encore. We listened, enchanted. How we had all missed the strangely comforting sound of a songbird!

At dusk my wife dropped on us all our grave responsibilities neglected: The Burial of Flutterball. I groaned and momentarily regretted suggesting interment under our tallest backyard rosebush. Once I found the shovel in the dimming twilight, I joined the party of bereaved in the backyard. While the kids stood around me, I dug the hole under wind-jostled pink blossoms. Timarie held a cardboard box that seemed a bit large for the hole.

"Why don't we forget the box?" I suggested, not wanting to dig up any more lawn to get a fit.

"You think so?"

"Yes."

The Last Menagerie

Timarie opened the box, folded back a wrap of white paper to reveal a small cloth shroud. She opened it with a sob and took a last look at our fallen yellow friend, stiff in death. Then she wrapped him again and placed him in the hole.

"Dear God, thanks for giving us Flutterball," Timarie prayed in a voice racked with sighs and sobs.

Nine-year-old Madeleine, putty-heart first class, began weeping. That cued twelve-year-old Molly into loud lamentation. And the three of them triggered little Franz, all of five years, into blubbering that seemed to spring from bewilderment. I stood silently and stoically by, as is the custom of the males in my line, rendered numb, even stupid, by death and its immediate effects. I wanted this painful rehearsal over with and to be back in the La-Z-Boy, where I could lose myself in a Bruin-Stanford basketball game with the PAC Ten title on the line.

Timarie invited the kids to pray, but they were occupied with bawling and couldn't get any words out.

"Let's all help bury him," Timarie said after I had covered the shroud with the first shovelful of dirt. Each took her or his turn filling the grave. I finished it off with four scoops that I patted down to the level of the lawn.

Marie eyed our labors with what seemed disapproval.

"I did all that to teach them about...prepare them for death," my wife informed me later that evening.

That she had, again. And again, I loomed the most likely candidate for the next mourning. Maybe that's why I felt so depressed.

What positive thing could I take from this modest tragedy? Well, if my wife tends me in *my* final days with the same comforting attention Flutter got, I will make that detestable transition in an envelope of love and care. (I just hope she doesn't bring in a new male the day after I'm planted.)

Memoirs of a Geezer Dad

The following day I found an old brass teakettle bearing a single lily and a solitary red rose atop Flutter's backyard grave; the kids had come up with a thoughtful makeshift monument.

Marie, the bird-killer, the realist, circled it, looking very thwarted. I sympathized with her, too.

Through luck and craft I managed to put off getting a family dog for a dozen years. It wasn't that I disliked dogs. Quite the contrary. But remembering the hands-on death-watch of my beloved Prunella, the Lab-Dalmatian mix from whom I knew no greater love, gave me much pause. And I knew from my first round of parenting that, despite all the promises I would hear from my children about how they would work around the clock taking care of the pooch, I would become the default dog-walker and pooper-scooper-upper when we got it. Speaking straight, I was too old and tired for anything bright and bothersome.

The luck I mentioned had to do with my wife. She was one of those few Americans who grew up without ever having a dog in the house. While she knew she had missed something, she wasn't quite sure how to fill the void. For one thing, she insisted that when we did get a dog it would have to be a vizsla—a choice the kids were cool to, favoring a Lab or golden retriever. Playing the skinflint card, I groaned over the high price of such an exotic breed. Stalemate. Stuck in committee–darn!

Then love jumped right in and broke the jam. My mother-in-law's bitch Molly, a black Lab/chow mix, became enamored of a pure-bred chocolate Lab next door, dug under the fence for one night of romance. The illegitimate issue included eight surviving pups that seemed to have observed Mendel's law: six black, two blond, and no chocolate brown at all.

The Last Menagerie

My animal midwife wife, on call the morning after the birth, held the littlest one—a black female with freckles on her belly—in her shirt's breast pocket and lost her heart immediately and completely. Visions of vizslas danced right out of her head. Charles Schulz was right; happiness is a warm puppy, especially when its eyes are still closed. Then and there tiny Mimi Rose became the unanimous choice for our first dog, to be picked up once she reached eight weeks and could leave her mother.

On that appointed dog-day afternoon, a warm and sunny Sunday, two of my oldest sons accompanied us in our raid on the litter. My oldest son Eric and girlfriend Anne took the dominant male, the big, blond brute Fred. My third son Karl and his wife Aliki chose the well-formed black Max, handsome with his chest star of white on the coat of coal. Of course, we loaded up our tiny trembling Mimi, and then the lot of us caravanned to our place for a spaghetti and meatball dinner and much good feeling.

After the pup-snuggling and a hectic photo shoot in which Mimi posed for pix with brothers Fred and Max, it was time for wobbly dogs and nervous owners to go their separate ways—or in my case remind myself that with the joy of addition came greater exposure to expensive vets and unpleasant backyard clean-up duties.

Life shifted into a higher state of mostly happy uproar. Mimi got a mixed reception—affectionate handling from the kids, the cold shoulder from Marie, who perceived early her status slip within the family. When the bemused pup approached the cat, Marie would launch a right-left paw combination to the snout that put you in mind of Sugar Ray Robinson. Why couldn't we all just get along? Well, later maybe.

Mimi proved easily housebroken. On the negative side of the ledger, she got teething relief by chewing on moldings,

Memoirs of a Geezer Dad

walls, furniture legs. And she inherited the Lab breed's passion for digging up backyard flowerbeds, which I replanted on a near-daily basis as part of my geezer exercise regimen.

"She needs obedience school," my wife ruled.

"I suppose," I said, hoping I was beyond draftable age.

I was relieved when Timarie herself took Mimi to Puppy Kindergarten for eight weeks of Thursday nights at the local recreation center. On the last Thursday she brought home the dog and a diploma with "pass" written next to her "Obedience Test Score." That the "Awarded High Honors for _____" line remained blank left me suspicious—even after my wife coaxed Mimi through a few "Sit" and "Stay" demonstrations for me.

"Your turn to take her to first grade," she instructed.

I wanted to balk, but didn't know how to do so without seeming a slacker.

Reluctantly and innocently, I showed up at the community center with pup, leash, and lead rope in hand. I nearly got jerked out of my shoes as Mimi attacked a well-behaved Chesapeake Bay retriever. I managed to restrain her and tug her into an orientation room where our instructor called roll ("a Lab mix," she said to herself as she checked Mimi's name off—the tone slightly demeaning, I thought). Then she accepted our checks. Sad to admit, the garrulous Mimi barked more than any of the score of mutts and bluebreds about to embark on their great learning experience. The instructor, who was having much difficulty making herself heard above the dog din, earned some sympathy and gratitude from me when she led us outside to a large expanse of concrete where the serious training was to begin. How did she keep her patience and poise working daily in doggie bedlam?

"Let's start with the command 'stay,'" she suggested. All

dogs obeyed their owners, except one. Mimi lunged in three of the four directions to make contact with her classmates. Her intentions were not honorable.

"Sit," we next said on command and in unison. All the canines got around to obeying, except for Mimi, who ran tight circles around me until the leash bound my ankles together. Sit could have been "anchored in place" as far as I was concerned.

Though I had judiciously stationed myself on the periphery of the great square (the better to not be seen), my shame and Mimi's disruptive antics were to go on for another 20 minutes.

The crisis came when the order was given to let our dogs lead us by the long rope. Twenty-one humans and their obedient canines walked south together. Mimi lunged north, trying to join a pick-up game on the adjacent, north-side basketball court.

The trainer approached me. "You know, I don't think she's as advanced as the other dogs," she said charitably. "You can have your check back…. I think it would be better if you put her in Puppy Kindergarten."

I was too embarrassed to say she'd already completed that training with my wife, and we had the document to prove it.

Instead, I took the returned check and put my figurative tail between my legs, yanking leash-tethered Mimi toward the car. My last vision of obedience school was of one of those wall-eyed terriers giving us both the stink-eye.

"You dunce!" I hissed when we reached the car, at a loss for a better word.

She cowered, lowered her tail in what I fancied false or short-lived contrition.

"You're back already?" my wife asked when we reached home.

"Permanently."

"What happened?"

Memoirs of a Geezer Dad

"She didn't obey a single command—she flunked out!"

I could tell she was about to give me the "there-are-no-bad-dogs, only-inept-masters" speech, then read my rage and wisely thought better of it.

I kept the peace, too. I didn't ask her how she finagled the diploma. Did they have crib notes? Or did they just buy the phony sheepskin?

Humiliating! Members of my household do not "flunk out." I was a full professor, for God's sake!

In a matter of days I learned that the idle paws of drop-out pups are the devil's workshop and point the little dears on the road to ruin. I had suspected Mimi of petty thievery before—hot dogs vanished from a kid's plate when a head was turned, cubes of margarine mysteriously disappeared from kitchen counters while I busied myself about my culinary duties.

But nothing approaching Grand Theft Chicken.

The little woman had to work late so I thought I'd reward her with a new chicken dish—boneless breasts soaked in a Thai marinade and served with a side of Oriental noodles…from the package, to be sure. (A house geezer can only be so gourmet.)

After taking the dish from the oven and setting it atop the kitchen counter, I tried a bite. Exquisite. Then I left the room to touch base with the falling Angels and their televised baseball game.

When my wife got home I returned to the kitchen to serve dinner. Gone. All four of the succulent Thai beauties, no longer swimming in marinade, had vanished from the Pyrex dish. It had been a stretch, but Mimi was a healthy pup and had grown into it, able to rear up and extend her neck into the middle of the counter top and gulp down all four breasts.

"You little bitch!" I bellowed.

Mimi looked away, feigning innocence at first, then rolled over on her back to expose her distended belly and doubly betray her guilt. Hopes for an Asian spice intolerance momentarily traversed my mind. But such vengeance could also mean a messy clean-up.

"They were really tasty," I told my wife.

She didn't find it in herself to compliment me.

Only a day later my second son Kurt brought me a loaf of freshly baked banana bread—a favorite of mine. Again I carelessly left it on the kitchen counter, set farther back, in the safety zone, I thought.

A return from calling the kids to dinner proved I was wrong. The rectangular loaf was transformed into a three-dimensional trapezoid—extra moist on its newly sheared side.

Two days in a row! From bad to worse. Damned delinquent! And another growth spurt promising even more spectacular future heists.

The third day I settled on a plan of revenge. At dinnertime I semi-carelessly left a loaf of *jalapeño* bread—adorned with a plump green mouth torch—on the counter within snout's reach. As I left the room she watched me, then passed me, doing her usual casual skulking. Just try it!

I returned ten minutes later. What? There was the *jalapeño* bread, untouched. There was the black Lab pup, eyeing me in her sly way. She didn't bite.

Then and there I had to change my opinion of Mimi. I could no longer consider her mentally deficient. It's all a matter of where you channel what smarts you're given. In fact, it was clear she had a first-rate criminal mind.

Though the thievery has continued to this day, Mimi and I have come to an understanding. As my children have dutifully explained to me time after time, if I'm stupid enough to leave food within her ever expanding reach, it's my fault, not hers; she's only acting out of instinct and can't control her natural drives.

Memoirs of a Geezer Dad

Mimi's most recent caper amused them to no end, and informed me again of how complex the simplest of events in life can be. Mimi had slithered up and scarfed half a can of warmed corned beef hash straight from the skillet while I left the kitchen for maybe 30 seconds. The kids call the product—Hormel's or Libby's or whatever the label—"Dad's dog-food" after its appearance. How fitting then that a dog should take its share! I was of course bummed to lose the treat. On the positive side, though, what I didn't eat was a processed, high-cholesterol product clearly not good for me. Then again, I had fetched it from the dented can bin and paid only 41 cents—a thrifty lunch any way you cut it. Go figure.

Ironically, time, place and circumstance have made close companions of Mimi and me; indeed, my children insist that I have become her favorite in the family. That's because when my wife's at work and the children are off to school we have only each other—to clean the kitchen together, to watch the stock market gyrations on CNBC together, and to take our constitutionals together. My only complaint concerns the walks, when her vigorous tugging on the leash so vigorously grinds my arthritic left hip joint to where I want to cry out in pain. I will need an artificial ball-and-socket replacement if I live much longer.

I confess I often regret the geezer shut-in's lonely life and long again for the workaday world, with its cast of friends, competitors, schemers, villains, thudheads and drones. To think that the guy who once interviewed presidential candidate John F. Kennedy on the steps of Royce Hall and took writer's junkets to Paris first class on Charles De Gaulle's centime now pet-sits for a servile living....

The Last Menagerie

And yet...Sartre said that all men are more than they seem. The same is true of animals. Bound to them by the rhythms of daily life, you form relationships with them, just as they do with each other; we find ourselves cast with them in real life's fleeting daily dramas that unfold around us in all their wondrous complexity.

The latest episode in "Further Adventures in Domesticity" casts me as referee in the ongoing saga of dog versus cat in the kitchen. This day they vie again for the leftover scraps caught in the seam of the tuna can. Nimble Marie gets to it first and gets an ecstatic lick in. But here comes the heavyweight wearing the black coat and with domination on her mind. Marie fires a lightening string of right jabs—should be leading with her left!—right into Mimi's eye-level fur. Oh no! Not a trip to the vet for an eye transplant! But not to worry.... Mimi brushes aside the blows and seizes the can as if she owns it, with no obligation to share. Labrador has won Round 43 in the Great Tuna War. Maybe tomorrow I'll rig the match in Tabbyland's favor by putting the can high on the counter. I have that power.

Meanwhile, our parade of pets has a new addition—another canary, unwanted and needing a home, rescued by none other than Timarie. The bird comes with the name Pete Koiheart Lustigvogel and is dominantly orange with a brown crown and a few white feathers toward the tail (like a koi fish)—an altogether handsome fellow, trimmer than Carmine

Memoirs of a Geezer Dad

and, I must admit, a more willing minstrel than our resident tenor and endowed with an equally fine voice.

For the time being, to head off any hurt feelings that might inhibit song, he will bunk far away from Carmine, with my bride and me in the master bedroom.

I hope he likes KUSC and dies before me. Let me amend that. I have outlived one dog, one cat, one canary and more goldfish than you can flush down a toilet. Among my living charges I have one dog and one cat and two canaries, and I intend to outlive them all. May it be so.

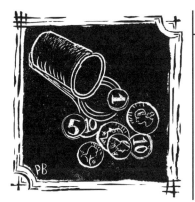

Chapter 6

(Chen You're No Longer 64

Folks like to make much of the fortieth year as life's major milestone, after which the good times are gone, and one's prospects gradually dim. But 65 is the big one, the defining one, when even the government takes notice and puts you on the Social Security and Medicare rolls. It's official. You're certified, in writing, in Washington, D.C., a Senior Citizen…or in my case, one glum geezer.

I dreaded my sixty-fifth birthday for all the obvious reasons and one that chance and the State of California conspired to add. It was the day my driver's license had to be renewed. As a reward for my good driving record, I had been favored with a decade's re-registrations by mail, but for this one I had to show up in person at the DMV and be tested.

It's my nature to take tests seriously, which may account for my waking to a nasty, painkiller-resistant gout attack the week before my birthday. After the morning's drudgery of getting breakfasts and lunches made and homework signed and wife and kids off to work and school, I called for an appointment.

"January 22. Go to Window 20, 9:10 a.m….sharp," the lady told me, rather brusquely. The pain not withstanding, I forced myself to make a trial drive to the DMV office with two purposes in mind. One, I wanted to time the driving distance to be sure I wasn't late to these difficult-to-get appointments. Second, I wanted to pick up the digest to the

Memoirs of a Geezer Dad

Motor Vehicle Code so I could review for the written test; failing to pass it would bring shame on me on my first day as a certified Senior Citizen and no doubt leave me without a license for a crucial time.

The trip took 23 minutes. And the digest that would refresh my knowledge of the rules of the road ran to 94 pages in the English version. (I don't know how many pages the Korean version ran, because I sheepishly returned it to the rack after I realized my mistake.)

Still ailing, I stopped on the way home to pick up my daughter Madeleine at her gymnastics class.

"Are you Timarie's father?" a woman who apparently knew my wife asked.

I have been mistaken as my children's grandfather too many times to count, and I've learned to roll with that punch. But this was the first time I had been misidentified as my wife's father.

Initially, I was shocked. "Yes," I said stupidly before recovering. "No, I mean I'm her husband."

The woman skillfully disguised her embarrassment and managed to avoid my eyes for the balance of my daughter's lesson. I found myself spiraling down into a deeper depression.

When I got home I consulted the mirror. No doubt about it, as they say in sports announcing. Age had snowed white hairs on me. My eyebrows had tripled their hair diameters, thereby defying the laws of gravity and grooming. The ear fuzz had become a tangled savanna. Alas, what I saw in the glass confirmed what I had seen in the just-developed last-Christmas photos where a geekish, graying, thin-haired guy wearing my noble chin stared uncomfortably back at me. I was old and getting older—fast.

Was there time to get a facelift before the driver's test?

When You're No Longer 64

Could I afford it?

How could I possibly show that face at my wife's fast-approaching twentieth high school reunion, where I was likely to be mistaken for her *grandfather*?

Did I dare stay at home?

Get the facelift whatever the cost?

I decided to concentrate on my mind instead. I put in at least ten hours of home study, cramming as I hadn't since college days. I tried all manner of mnemonic devices to impress on my tired old mind the facts they would expect me to know...such as the recurrence of fives in the digit column for speed limits: 65 mph for freeways, 25 mph for school zones, 15 mph for vision-obstructed railroad crossings. And so on.

On the appointed morning I left home with a ten-minute cushion of time that I might spend in the parking lot going over blood-alcohol levels—of only academic interest to this abstainer, though they wouldn't know that. I even filled out a form in advance that updated my vital statistics: hair color from brown to gray; height the same six feet, four inches, but the weight up 20 pounds from the svelte motorist I used to be.

At 9:08 I stepped up to Window 20. I was asked to sign the register and then step back behind the floor line and wait my turn for Window 22, where a middle-aged woman with a bored mechanical half-smile was taking a personal check from a patron. I would probably be next. So far, so good. My eyes strayed to a modest-sized sign to my right:

"Cash, checks, and money orders only."

What? No plastic! I live on credit card float!

Panic entered the room...or at least my mind. I dragged my wallet out and opened the proper section. Eleven dollars. It cost ten dollars, didn't it? I seemed to remember that.

"Next."

I stepped forward. "This is where I pay?"

Memoirs of a Geezer Dad

"Yes it is."

"How much is the fee?"

"Fifteen dollars."

"I've forgotten my checkbook."

Her face was sympathetic, but unyielding.

"I only have 11 dollars cash."

Her head moved from side to side. "It's 15 dollars."

"Well, would you save my place? I'll go to the car and check...my parking change."

She shrugged.

Flustered, I searched all the crannies of my wallet enroute to the car. Perhaps I had stashed a fiver somewhere as I sometimes do. No, but I did find a dollar bill folded into the size of a postage stamp. A spark of hope. That made 12 dollars...just three to go.

I took my spark to the car. I periodically fill three little 35mm photo canisters to the non-rattling brim with a mix of coins for parking meters, emergency phone calls, and such. Unfortunately, they seldom survive for long the periodic raids by my two young daughters on what amounts to their unsanctioned petty cash fund. I make a practice of scattering the three canisters. One goes in the recess under the radio for easy-access. A second goes into the glove compartment behind the hand towels. My final cartridge, the hidden reserve, is cleverly stashed in the map drawer under the shotgun seat.

Once in the car I reach under the radio well. Empty. Even the cartridge cap is missing. The vandals had passed by here. Disheartening, but not the end of the world. It's the propitiatory offering, after all—what the grave-robbers were supposed to find, protection money...whatever.

I thrust my hand into the glove compartment and draw out number two. It rattles...and it shouldn't if it were full, as I had left it. My stomach churns as I spill out the contents on the seat. No quarters. Just dimes, nickels, pennies. So they skimmed off the gravy!

I can't make it without quarters! Downright agitated, I pull the final rattling canister from under the seat, rip off the cap and roll out its contents as though they were dice in life's biggest crapshoot. A quarter! No, on closer inspection it was a bogus look-alike, from the Shell Famous Facts and Faces Game, Alexander Graham Bell being the worthy honoree.

Well, at least they had been merciful and pretty much left the lesser denominations. With trembling fingers I started my counting and stacking...only one quarter left...but 11 dimes...23 nickels...43 pennies. That made...$14.93! Oh no! Seven cents shy!

Back to the window I hurried. What could I do? I would look pitiable and helpless. (No great effort there.) Her heart would melt, and she would say, "I'll give you the seven cents." Slight emphasis on the "give" so I knew it wasn't a loan, and of course such a piddling sum would not have to be paid back.

The lady at the window made no such offer. Just gave me the mechanical half-smile. "I'm sorry," she said unconvincingly, but with finality.

"Can I go home...and come back later today?"

"Yes, but you'll have wait for an opening."

I groaned, softly, but audibly. That would probably stretch my stay there into the mid-afternoon.

I thought of pasting on a smile and singing to my fellow motorists, "Brother, can you spare a dime." But I knew it wouldn't fly in such a humorless place as the DMV. Besides, it just is not in me, as it wasn't in my father before me, or my two brothers. Pride, whatever, doesn't allow us to ask for donations (even directions, for that matter).

Memoirs of a Geezer Dad

"Will you hold my place for just five more minutes?" I pleaded.

She looked around and saw her next client proceeding slowly. "I'll do my best."

I rushed into the parking lot again on a search-and-destroy mission. I spotted no coins on the asphalt, but when I got to the minivan I quickly ripped up the front floor mat and there it was, shiny still among the beach sand and boot-dirt: a dime! Hallelujah! I had $15.03!

Back at the window, I confidently, and somewhat resentfully, pushed the ten and the one and all my accumulated coins across the counter top. The woman methodically counted them out and pushed back three pennies. I was tempted to say, "Keep the change for your troubles," but I'm too timid for that.

"Take this to Window 11," she said, handing me my paperwork.

I moved in that direction, no doubt where I would take my written test.

"Step back to the line," the young Asian man said after accepting my forms and receipt.

I did.

"Now read the top two lines on the chart," he instructed.

Done. No problem for this farsighted geezer. The young man did his sorting and stamping of my papers and handed them back.

I waited. He looked questioningly at me. "Yes?"

"Do I take the driving test here? The written test?"

He smiled, rather kindly, but indulgently as well. "You don't have to take that test. You're done."

Was I ever! Overdone and smoking! The great progressive State of California doesn't accept Visa for payment and no longer tests its senior citizens on the rules of the road! Some kind of mixed priorities. And I was never told either.

70

When You're No Longer 64

I was still simmering about the many hours wasted studying when I merged onto the San Diego Freeway and almost immediately heard the thump-thump of a tire or tires in distress. Mine! Oh, no! Sounded like the right front. Miles from home and with three cents in my pocket! Did I continue to drive and hope to make it home and ruin the six-month-old tire?

Wait! Wasn't this section of the San Diego Freeway where they scored the pavement and your tires sounded like they were flat but they really weren't? Maybe, but I couldn't remember, and in any case I'd better ease over to an off-ramp and off the freeway—at the cost of a good tire, if that had to be.

Offramps proved scarce on this particular stretch of the San Diego, and I sweated out nearly two miles of deceleration with hopes of finding a surface street service station before my rims were squared and I came to a grinding halt.

Eureka! There it was! A Mobil station at the foot of the ramp! And I had a Mobil card, which they would certainly accept.

I got out of the car. I stared. All the tires were fine. So it *was* the pavement. No need to buy a tire. Or use my card to buy any gas, for that matter. What gratitude I felt was offset by a new shame. Befitting my age, I got back in and drove slowly and carefully home, feeling a great physical relief when I turned the ignition off in my driveway. At least no one I knew had witnessed my solo clown act.

I had survived my rite of passage, but in a diminished state, simultaneously wiser and dumber than I was when I was 64. Knowing more about the California Motor Vehicle Code than any sixty-five-year-old in captivity was small compensation. The greater lesson learned was that I now know senescence does not creep up on you at the petty pace of month to month, but comes all at once, on the day you turn 65.

As for the future, I've refilled the photo canisters and issued

Memoirs of a Geezer Dad

stern anti-theft warnings (and hid yet a fourth under the driver's seat). I'm also thinking of having coins sewn into the waistband of my Dockers, along with an identification patch of who I am and where I live and the phone number of a responsible party.

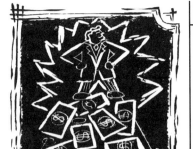

Chapter 7

A Small Fortune Come and Gone

Iᴛ's ɴᴏᴛ ᴛʜᴀᴛ I ever had anything against money. It's just that I wasn't up to doing what was necessary to get it. It's not that I preferred a fairly Spartan existence for me and my get, but that is the consequence of always living in the present and working as a journalist and then a teacher. At least that's how I rationalize living a life—and inflicting such a life on my loved ones—that was pretty must salary-financed month to month.

For a time I wasn't even aware that I wasn't keeping up with the Joneses. Or the Smiths. Or the Browns. The future? It would be there for me, waiting to be claimed with a best-selling novel or hitting the Pick Six at Santa Anita. But as I progressed through my mid-thirties, I began to notice that my contemporaries who were engaged in more financially rewarding lines of work pulled ahead of me in better cars, left me behind in marginal neighborhoods, and provided things for their children that I never could provide for mine.

Savings? Not much left after the day-to-day expenses of raising three kids. Investments? I had only two brushes with the stock market: One in the early 1970s had been a short and bloody fleecing at the hands of a Merrill Lynch broker skilled in the art of churning in a static market; the other was a modest sum put in a growth mutual fund that slept for ten years, and when I cashed it in I had made all of $60. Bad karma? No, bad market timing was my problem, or so a wise broker later told me.

The "investments" I preferred back in those carefree days

ran to such consumer non-durables as beer, wine, gin, and excursions to Hollywood Park, where the five-dollar window proved an exciting rat-hole. Foolish, to be sure. But then it seemed as good a place as any for not-quite-discretionary dollars—if you were looking for some excitement. So it meant living as a financially marginal man…that life was exhilarating.

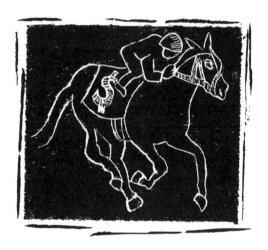

Then I hit my mid-forties, suddenly divorced, sharing custody of my three young sons, living from paycheck to paycheck that went mostly for rent, embarked on an exciting new low-paying career as a lecturer in journalism at California State University Long Beach. Chastened, I got serious. Worked harder. Climbed the promotion ladder to tenured full professor and met my second wife, a student, in a covert romance that never quite made it to scandal status. For a brief window of time I was content being the oldest living bohemian in Huntington Beach with his original set of teeth and a roof over his head.

Then came the second wave of children, taking the places of the three who left. Daughter, daughter, accidental son

A Small Fortune Come and Gone

arrived in three-year intervals. My days of living near the poverty line had to end. My luck had to change. And my time to change it was running out.

Necessity is an unlikely mom. After paying off my divorce lawyer and settling my debts with house sale proceeds, we invested the remaining $20,000 in a small business that seemed to have bright prospects. Turns out it did, returning $62,000 in profit after three years. When we cashed out we set aside money for our young children's future education—UTMAs at Fidelity Investments, the money put in its Growth and Income fund. Those mutual funds waxed steadily if unspectacularly during the mid-1990s.

With my own modest Keogh Plan and a couple of piddling IRAs, I got more daring. I subscribed to Value Line, watched CNBC daily, opened a brokerage account, signed up to trade on margin, then plunged into tech stocks for "one of the great bull market rides of all time." I watched with a raw chump's awe my stocks soar and split, soar and split, then do it all again. Wow! Payback, after all those years of just scraping by as a salary slave! It was all so sudden, all so effortlessly easy!

My wife thought I'd turned into some kind of financial genius. I didn't dare go that far. Luck—in the way of market timing—as much as skill figured in my success, I knew, but I did feel my hubris swelling, the way changing a roadside flat made an apprentice of me in the company of master mechanics. Maybe I should take the slow-growing kids' funds and move them into high tech, too? Something to think about.

Three months before I turned 65, I appeared, as notified by mail, at my local Social Security office. As instructed, I

75

Memoirs of a Geezer Dad

brought my birth certificate, discharge papers, marriage certificate, latest IRS tax forms, and W2s. I admit I felt nervous, even sensed a little dread rising from within. With the exception of popping in for a passport now and again, I hadn't been in a federal government office since June 8, 1956, when I walked out of Manhattan Beach Air Force Station, Brooklyn, New York, with my honorable discharge in hand, free at last. There were all those stories about red tape and bureaucracy and such.

My fears proved groundless. The young woman who had my file open on her desk was courteous, deliberate, thoughtful. Amazing! She opened my entire record of working for a living—going back to the Restoration Period—before our very eyes. Only my days as a paperboy were missing. That said, there wasn't much in dollars and cents to show for it, really. (The non-material seeker of truth had not accumulated as many credits as you might think. Take heed, all ye liberal arts majors!)

Then the young woman began talking about the $300 a month each of my children would be receiving from Social Security.

"Pardon me," I interrupted, "but I don't plan on dying over the next three months."

She smiled warmly. "No, these are not survivor benefits. Just benefits."

Slow dawn for this benighted senior. "You mean they get money just because I'm 65?"

"Yes, because they are minor children. While the money will come to you, it must go toward their welfare, of course. You understand?"

"Of course. Like, say, putting it away in a college education fund?"

"That would be perfect."

A Small Fortune Come and Gone

Wonderful! Becoming an official geezer had some hidden benefits I hadn't figured on. Of course it made very good social sense, though I doubted my legions of Republican neighbors would see it that way.

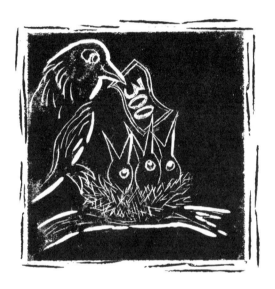

"Thank *you!*" I burbled to the young woman, as though she were personally responsible for this windfall. She smiled again, comfortable with heroine status, however undeserved. I left the office feeling pretty good about the future of my children and my country; dealing with the Feds wasn't nearly as traumatic as my fellow Orange Countians like to have you believe.

I happily report that I dithered over moving the children's UTMAs into brokerage accounts where I could wheel and deal their futures in the market. I unhappily report that I stayed the course with my Keogh and IRAs and rode the bull right over the cliff, also known as the tech wreck. With the crash of 2000–2002 I was suitably humbled even as the long-time masters of Wall Street, wise in the ways of diversification

77

Memoirs of a Geezer Dad

and short-selling, survived reasonably intact. In 18 months the man of means became the man of little means once more, with too many shares of World Com, Lucent, JDS Uniphase and Tyco in his brokerage accounts. Strangely, I was not as depressed as I thought I might be, but felt almost comfortable at being restored to normalcy. That smug, grinning guy with the swollen portfolio was never me. No, I'm the sweating old fellow out front behind the lawnmower, the only guy left on his block who still cuts his own front lawn.

My fig leaf as our family financial advisor is that I never did put my children's savings accounts into go-go growth stocks. Funds enough remain to pay their ways through a decent college, which is where the life worth living begins anyway.

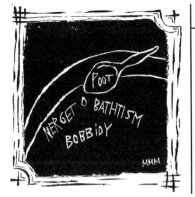

Chapter 8

House
of
Words

PROBABLY BY GENES more than choice or chance, ours is a word family. We worship words for far more than their utilitarian value. Sure, we use them in daily discourse as journalists do to inform each other with the famous five Ws—who, what, where, when, and why. And in a tip of the cap to our material, self-indulgent age, we add a sixth "W" for want, as in "I want a new bat" or "I want a new blouse."

More importantly, though, we treasure the spoken word and the written word for their entertainment value—particularly the humor they make possible. Lastly, we prize words for their intrinsic worth and their power to edify when strung together meaningfully and musically, as in poetry.

How does this translate into daily family life? *Noisily* would be the adverb. *Play* would be the noun. Each member is encouraged to blurt out anything that comes to mind...or does it even without encouragement. One has carte blanche to be silly or theatrical. Each is allowed—even if reluctantly—to try out new foreign accents or relapse into baby talk. Echolalia is always welcome. Puns are exalted. Nonsense rules.

Of course, when you get enough mouths open and yammering, things can get out of hand. That's when we use words to a fault, talking over and through one another, until the verbal din sends me scurrying off seeking silent refuge from the layered babble.

Memoirs of a Geezer Dad

My wife and I are both carriers of the talky gene. But I'm the primary culprit when it comes to passing along its more extreme, obsessive traits. For 37 years I've been collecting the utterances of my six kids as though they were rare butterflies, jotting them down in my journals, a precious collection I can always go back to for nourishing memories.

Language for me is a boundless playground where anything goes. The sheer wonder of it—this evolutionary gift of symbols first heard and then written down as abstractions of abstractions—that makes us the remarkable, self-aware species we are. Words, after all, lead us to the discovery of beauty and our own mortality and allow us to pass on to generations unborn what we've thought and how we've felt.

If there's anything I love more than language it's listening to my children acquire it, or better yet, butchering it with their own youthful inventions that come and go like meteors in the night sky. If the blunder is especially funny or appealing, I'll steal it and, with the complicity of other family members, perpetuate with a straight face the malformed word in the family gab as long as I can.

Cruel? Maybe. But great fun...until I get caught, as was the case not long ago.

"If we're going to fix the Game Boy we'll need the destructions," I said to Franz. He gave me a chilly "forget-it" look.

Deserved. I had been caught again in my mocking game of using his malapropism as though it were the right word. He had coined "destructions" the previous Christmas when we started to assemble toys Santa had left. I seized on it as an unconscious improvement on "instructions," given how he treated his toys. Now he knew his mistake—and my deception.

Invariably, when children learn of their goofs, they are not amused. Indeed, they studiously avoid ever using the word or

pronunciation again, and give me an even colder stare if I try
to reroute them back to the "cute" old ways. They've been
duped and are unforgiving of their dupers.

I wistfully invoke these self-reminders to prepare myself for
Franz outgrowing the age of blunder. "Destructions" will now
go to the dead-word bin to join such Franz creations as Nerget
the Frog, resident with Hernie and Helmo on the *Sesame
Street* we used to watch together. I know my pickings will
dwindle to nothing soon, and my journal will be the less for it.

The prospect saddens me, and at the same time heartens
me with the realization that words outlive those who use
them. That may account for these very words and why I write
them down, with future readers close to me in mind. I feel no
guilt, however, for the word games I play at my children's
expense. And if I did, I doubt I could change a thing.

To chart the pathology of my word-hoarding habits, I
recently sought out my oldest son, Eric, whose crib I stood
beside in the spring of 1966, an excited first-time father waiting
for his first word so I could write it down. I asked him if he
remembered that his first three syllables strung together were
"Doo-nee-na." Of course he did, because I was so enamored of
the sound that I adopted "dunina" on the spot and have used it
ever since as a synonym for a gizmo, or thingamabob, or do-
hickey when I can't recall a noun's real name. Eric looked
away; seemed he took no pride in authorship.

"Of course that's not a real word," I said. "Your first real
word was actually 'Noumea'…say, how did you know the capital of New Caledonia at two months?" Eric saw no humor in
the fact that his three syllables fell into meaningful sequence by
mere chance, and I took them at ear's value. Rather, he looked

pained, having a hard time humoring an aging father who was obviously losing it.

My second son Kurt was more a butcher than a coiner of words. My favorite was catching him at age five singing the Christmas carol line "Toll the ancient Yuletide carol" as "Troll the aged you'll fight Carol." I like to observe each Christmas season by dredging that one up in his presence, not failing to explain to others that his baby-sitter at the time was named Carol, and he was an avid fisherman from the word go. So there was a semilogical explanation for the gaffe after all. His smile is weak, indulgent.

Kurt's twin brother Karl approached language more carefully and uttered aloud fewer keepers. Still, he gave us "kwakwee" for water, and that got a few years of life. More enduring was "Catoween" for Halloween—a word that lives on in the current household, thanks exclusively to my heroic efforts at preservation.

Karl's sweet-toothed half-sister Madeleine has made valuable contributions as well. While still in her high chair, she came up with "bobbidy" for banana and "Mamady" for "Mama give me." Mamady bobbidy—that mellifluous blend of assonance and consonance earned a proud place in our family lexicon, even when our appetite for bananas soured. To this day, when the bobbidies go brown and soft and draw fruit flies to the bowl, someone is apt to say, "looks like it's time for bobbidy bread." Madeleine gave us another word that has become a family mainstay. She was four and in her car seat as the family headed home on the freeway when she asked aloud, "Are we in Sayman Beach yet?" Sayman...for Huntington? The stretch was so great and the linkage so obscure that we all fell in love with Sayman immediately, and to this day it is an oft-used synonym for home.

Molly, my first daughter and oldest child of my second family, is probably the most verbal of my children and the best coiner of new words. (My wife takes some credit for that, believing that her reading aloud Joyce's *Dubliners* while nursing the newborn set her down the verbal path; who am I to disagree?)

Molly's the one who at age three, as we drove by the Wilmington, California, launch pad for the Goodyear blimp, observed, "There's the New Year bloop." I swallowed my mirth and successfully perpetuated the family use of "New Year bloop" for nearly a year. Then she learned of her error, and I got my chilly look of rebuke.

What really amazes me about Molly is that, by my lights, the words she invents are often superior to the ones in use. Take her word "starberry" coined at age three for strawberry. Look down at the sepal that clings to the fruit. Is that a star or what? How much more appropriate than "straw" as a prefix!

She also came up with "scampion" for champion. For one who wins, but cuts a few corners in the process, I guess.

Or how about "bathtism" for the sacrament Baptism? What logic at work! Forget derivations! What an improvement!

Her most incisive neologism appeared at age two in "mortacycle" for motorcycle. She didn't even know that she had lost an uncle to one of those infernal machines when she was 18 months old.

I guess my favorite, though, remains "poot"—a three-year-old's multi-purpose noun/verb improvement on poop, covering excreta in its solid, gaseous and liquid states. As you might imagine, it has become the euphemistic coinage of convenience in our realm.

Given my neologistic obsession, and considering that I am keeper of the journal, it's no surprise that some of my own creations have become fixtures in the family lexicon. Most often used would be the word "brink" and its prolific family. It's the phonetic root of the Portuguese word "brincar" that I picked up

Memoirs of a Geezer Dad

in the Air Force in 1955, and means, as best as I could ever get a translation from the Portuguese troops I served with, goofing off, behaving lazily and stupidly.

Like any good, healthy verb (brink not, want not; or brink, brink, brink like you've never brinked before), it has grown a noun identity as well (brinker—one who brinks), and is to be found in gerund form as in "no brinking," not to mention compound noun service (as "brink zone" or "brink-out" or "brink camp"—a location where clutter from some abandoned fantasy rests curbside in plain, ugly view). It has even achieved compound adjectival status, as in "Let's declare this a brink-free day." Also useful and easy-to-mouth is brinkable, meaning something you can goof-off with, or brinkerette—a petite female goofer-offer. Twice now my children have encountered people with the surname "Brinker," and I have seen their mouths gape and jaws drop in stunned amusement.

My borrowings from the Portuguese do not end there, I'm obligated to say by way of an embarrassing confession. I've always marveled at parents who discipline their children in a calm voice and dispassionate manner. Those who bring sweet reason to misunderstandings and abuse their kids with words or blows not at all.

I marvel at them; I do not imitate them...unfortunately. Rubbed raw over a day of sibling spats and/or slob conduct, I can be quick to anger and over-long at making peace. To my credit, though, I rarely ever take my satisfaction physically, with a cuff or a smack delivered to an accessible limb or ham. Naturally, I use words. Angry words. Ironic words. Or, that failing, bad words.

While good old Anglo Saxon crudities are always preferred, using those self-satisfying, harsh consonantal sounds poses a few serious drawbacks. First, you're teaching your kids words you don't want them using. ("But you say 'bleep' all the time!" is

the common rejoinder.) Second, their very taboo nature pre-
vents you from using such words in public—unless you don't
mind the world at large knowing you hail from *la bas*.

What to do? Well, I found a solution early in raising my first
family of three boys born 15 months apart (also known as "my
time in diaper hell"). I cussed them out in Portuguese. This
linguistic windfall came of that same year's liaison duty abroad
with the Portuguese Air Force; while I learned very little proper Portuguese, I did manage to pick up about everything that
was crude and vulgar and, in some cases, impossible to really do,
if you took the words literally.

Those words my NATO buddies taught me and which I laid
on my first three boys had the lovely, trilly vowel sounds of a
song. My steam got released, the kids knew my state of mind,
and no one was the wiser for it, in public or in private.

During rare interludes of domestic peace my sons would ask
me what the words meant. They would even repeat them,
though fortunately with the pronunciation sufficiently distorted.

"I'll tell you when you're 18" was my concession to their
curiosity.

When they reached 18 as a herd and made the request
again, I stalled them. "When you're 21," I promised, hoping
they'd forget about them by then.

Not to be. So, with their maturities and peace made, I
translated all. They roared their laughter, savoring each vile
word in the litany that had become familiar music to their
young ears.

I returned to monolingualism with my second family.
Maybe it was because the first two were girls, and the old ways
and words just didn't seem appropriate somehow. Instead, I
employed irony, as in "You look exhausted—probably from all
the help you gave me cleaning the kitchen," said to a daughter who stood by and did nothing while I sweated out two

hours of toil. Or, "I hear the United Cockroaches of America have named you 'girl of the year' for turning your room into a housing project for homeless vermin."

Irony is supposed to be corrective. Trouble is, it's an acquired taste, and its subtleties often escape the young.

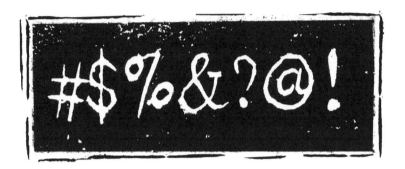

I confess that with the advent of Franz, my last child and last son, I've reverted on occasion to the "Portuguese Solution." In every case but one it happened when he was between two and four years old and had thrown one of his patented fits in a supermarket or department store. These would consist of a warning shriek or two, then his collapse on the store floor, where he would go limp with his unblinking blue eyes open and staring up into eternity. I was left standing next to the seemingly deceased child, struck down in the prime of his toddlerhood by a brutal and murderous parent, being glared at by loving mothers who weighed calling the police.

The first of these Fosbury Flops (as I came to call them, after the old Oregon high-jumper) occurred in a Lucky supermarket one day when two-year-old Franz decided to throw one because I had denied him a toy he wanted. As confounded as I was humiliated, all I could do was spin around, throw my limp bag-of-bones son over my shoulder, and march quickly out of the store without returning any stares, my half-filled shopping cart left behind for restocking. Sorry about that. Get the perishables before they melt or spoil.

The Flops ended one day when I simply left the four-year-old inert under a round rack of blouses in Mervyn's, feigning disgust at how some other parent's child was behaving.

I now realize his fits were less a reaction to not getting the toy he wanted than the early onset of the common male aversion to shopping—acute in his case. You might say that's easily remedied. Don't take him shopping. You would be right, and that's what I resolved to do.

Unfortunately, that's not always possible. Last spring I foolishly took both my baseball-playing son and softball-playing daughter to the sporting goods store for gear at the same time. That was my first mistake. Second mistake, I got Franz's cleats first, then began the search for daughter Molly's compression shorts and high socks. This, of necessity, takes more time. Since his needs were met, son Franz began reacting to the delay with an updated version of the Fosbury Flop that involved loud moaning and groaning and draping himself over several pieces of display furniture in protest.

Under such provocation, I reverted to the old ways. Out poured a truncated version of the Portuguese fusillade.

I heard a gasp and turned toward it. There she stood, about 35, with the brown hair, olive skin, slightly aquiline shape of nose, and narrow Mediterranean skull that I remembered seeing so often on Lisbon streets. Her look straddled shock and horror. In protective mode, she took a step between me and the young boy whose hand she held.

I didn't give her time to see my face redden. I yanked my kid by his arm and dragged him to a remote corner of the store until Molly met her needs on her own.

Memoirs of a Geezer Dad

This experience has left me chastened and resolved to speak no more Portuguese. Southern California has become just too cosmopolitan to get away with that kind of linguistic license any more. Young guttermouths are bad enough. But a geezer from the gutter? Not me.

Chapter 9

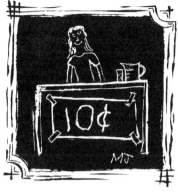

Careers in Progress

I WONDER WHAT MY youngest children will grow up to be. Not just in the broadest sense, the whole person formed by inner desire and outward circumstance. But what they will do for a living—their occupations. Why? Because I probably won't be around when they settle into their careers.

That's why I'm so very attentive to my kids' role-playing, and I monitor their fantasy lives for clues to what the future might bring them. I want to know and guide them if I possibly can.

Let me admit that I was not very good at prognosticating with my first family. My oldest son Eric, whom I projected as either a lawyer or a confidence man, given his argumentative nature and way of twisting words to suit his purposes, became a general contractor. (Some might find a synthesis there.) My son Kurt—he of the quick bat and rifle arm that I thought might be a major league baseball player—teaches literature and writing at a nearby community college. And Karl, the boy with a passion for music and guitars, whom I had pegged as a rock musician, owns a successful sculpture studio in Burbank that serves the entertainment industry.

With my second family, I hope to do better. To that end, since they were in preschool I've tracked their job aspirations through what I call "found documents."

Among this geezer dad's favorite things, found documents are my kids' writings and drawings—mostly works in progress—

Memoirs of a Geezer Dad

that advance some fantasy du jour. They will post them, then abandon them, and it will fall to me to dispose of them in the trash can, or retrieve them therefrom, or at least write down the contents of the no-longer-relevant memos, signs and posters. Call it sentimentality if you will. The second-time-around father wants to hold on to such things.

Preserve them, yes. For the self now, them later, perhaps. The one no-no is that I don't confront them with my discoveries...intrude on their fantasies with questions I might have. (That self-imposed rule may derive from having my own fantasy life mocked as a child.)

There are times when I want to meddle. Take my daughter Molly's first poem that I discovered and copied:

The Sheep's Wool.
When we cut sheeps' wool off
We make nice warm things like sweaters.
And when we make the sweaters in wintertime
The sheeps will be cold.
So why don't we put the sweaters
On the sheeps and be fair?

The eternal literature teacher in me wanted to critique and return: "Not very lyric; while the central idea is engaging, it raises the legitimate question, 'Then why shear them in the first place?'" But I didn't. That would be to intrude, spoil the spell.

A few months later I found a fragment written in her hand:
"Once upon a time, of the eyes of the owls and the swing of trees, and the breeze"

Right on! Lyric, yes! So like a born poet to catch the music of words and let the meaning catch up later. I wanted to tell her of the promise I saw in the fragment. But again, I restrained myself. Her world to inhabit…free of critics.

My favorite fantasy was The Detective Agency, begun by Molly but participated in by her younger sister Madeleine who joined the firm late. I confess to being baffled by the sign on their bedroom door:

THE SPY ROUT

OPEN AS ALWAYS

Were detectives and spies such close kin as to be inter-changeable? Just what was this "route" that was always open? To non-spies and non-detectives as well? They were forswear-ing their privacy? Nope. Not my business to ask.

Apparently the firm prospered, because it soon moved to slightly larger quarters in the computer room/study, a.k.a. Dad's writing room. I could see the advantages in the move. My soon-to-be-scattered office supplies were momentarily plentiful and at the agency's disposal. Up went a new sign:

WE SPY

YOU PAY 1 DOLLER AN-HOUR

DOCTER TOO

The fee seemed reasonable, but again I had questions. Was the medical practice a subsidiary of the spying operation? Spying being a sometime-dangerous profession, medical care seemed a logical spin-off. But did they bill separately? And if a spy got hurt in the line of work, did he or she get free medical care…or the kind of socialized medicine my right-wing con-gressman gets and stoutly denies to others?

91

Memoirs of a Geezer Dad

And just who was practicing medicine without a license? Madeleine, judging by a diagnosis I found written in her hand: **"Open sergery not inquired."** That was one patient saved, but how about the rest? Another unanswered question I will take to the grave.

Whim, or perhaps a malpractice suit, forced a career change. Molly and Madeleine next became fantasy educators of neighborhood kids, unfortunately using my writing room as both the principal's office and the classroom. The paperwork generated drove me crazy, and I couldn't find a thing I needed in the clutter of grade reports and stern notes to parents warning of their sons' and daughters' impending failures. Worst of all, they targeted their young brother Franz as class scapegoat, giving him straight Fs and repeatedly putting him "on detention." I almost broke my self-imposed silence. They should be building the little guy up, not tearing him down! But I bit my tongue and didn't. It was, after all, their trip.

I took the end of one semester as an opportunity to give my office its once-a-year cleaning. My excavation of the desk and floor of their educational paraphernalia filled two waste baskets to the brim. As I neared completion of my dig, I came across a document in Madeleine's hand that jolted me to attention:

The Knife is in the breefcase in the buganvea. The murder of Larry L. Meyer will be on 10/30/99.

P.S. Don't do anything to let them know.

OR else

Me! Intended victim of a murder conspiracy! My code of silence was momentarily broken. I went right into Madeleine's room and confronted her with the document. "Is this yours?" I asked.

"Yes," she admitted, not as guiltily as I would have liked.

"Well?"

An insinuating smirk was all I got.

"The date has passed...but am I still going to be murdered?"

"No," she said with a sly grin that told me the contract had expired with the fantasy.

I didn't ask her for any more details of the plot. Fantasies belong to those who spin them. As long as I was out of danger...and there was a detective in the house.

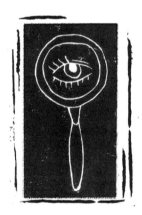

Like their father, all my children are incurable dreamers, fantasizers who drift through childhood imagining futures as famous novelists, Major League Baseball All-Stars or rock 'n' roll legends. Not for us the work-a-day world of business...no, just not constitutionally fit to toil for another in a conventional office.

Except for one. The mutant Madeleine. She's a fantasist like the rest of us...but her fancies are down-to-earth, money-minded, career-oriented, and often involve a redesign of our home into a specific place of business.

I spotted the anomaly when she was six, and I remember the spring day as though it were yesterday. She wanted to set up a juice stand on the front lawn so she could "make some money." No child of mine had ever made such a request before. Not wanting to discourage any such practical turn of mind, I caved in quickly to her usual relentless grindings. We live in a crass commercial age, I told myself. Wasn't it my duty to prepare her for the competitive business world that awaited her?

At her bidding, I opened a half-gallon of Welch's grape juice as she set up her stand. For it she commandeered an empty kennel box (usually used to incarcerate the cat) and a little wooden stool her late-grandfather had made especially for her. From the garage she fetched a stock of Dixie cups I didn't know we had, apparently abandoned by various insects as dry holes; she blew out the dirt that had settled in them. (Caveat all ye emptors.) She also dug out of some musty nook an old martini pitcher from my distant days of gin and roses, rinsed and filled it with juice and ice cubes, and hand-scrawled out her sign, "Cold Juice 10 sents." My heart turned to Jello. Right out of Norman Rockwell.

"We'll need more juice," she said after 20 minutes of inactivity.

"Why don't we wait until business picks up?" I responded. If you compared the number of potential sales at 10 cents each and what I paid for the grape juice, I wasn't sure I wanted it to.

Not to worry. Business was slower than slow. Stopped, in fact. At noon, after she'd spent two patient hours at the stand stroking the cat and searching the sidewalk for potential customers, I took her a lunch of cheese and crackers, which she could rinse down with her own stock. I also took out a dime.

"Can I buy a glass?"

She beamed and poured juice into a cup. (I took on faith that she'd blown out any spider poop.) As she turned to put the dime in her little and empty cash box, I spat out the juice behind my back. It didn't have the age and bite of the grape juice I'd reluctantly given up years before.

Ten minutes later she started looking restless. "I'm tired, Dad."

"You want to close down your juice stand?"

"Yes. It's boring."

"Yes, business often is."

"I'm going inside to color."

"Good idea," I said. "I'll close up shop for you." Maybe she'd grow up to be an artist, I thought. Pays about the same.

What I should have done was point out to her the reasons why the venture had failed...the lessons learned: First, find a demand before you mix up a supply. Second, choose a hot summer day rather than a cool and breezy spring day to sell cold drinks. Third, don't count heavily on sidewalk sales when you live on a frontage road. In sum, develop a good business plan to move product. (I think that's how MBAs talk.)

But I didn't. Why? Maybe I secretly wished she'd give up her entrepreneurial notions and rejoin the rest of our feckless lot of sandcastle-builders.

If that was my motive, I was misguided. Her drive only increased over the next four years as she operated, among other ventures, a private school, a cosmetics emporium, and a big-time corporate headquarters for a firm whose only business seemed to be ordering people about.

In itself laudable, I suppose. Except that she based her operations in Dad's writing room. My supplies became her supplies. My ever-diminishing space her ever-expanding space. Moreover, every change of fantasy involved an office redesign and fed her

Memoirs of a Geezer Dad

Aristotelian passion for pasting all the walls and appurtenances of her trade with labels—Avery's large chartreuse rectangles preferred—with names, numbers, or directions. And she never engaged a janitorial service.

One day, failing to find in the general mess a single pen of mine and all 19 pencils with broken points, I swallowed my rage and called an emergency family meeting. The children heard a semi-stern lecture on respect for others' property, most particularly my property. The mess was bad enough. The plunder was worse, and I wasn't going to take it anymore.

"There are nine canister-containers in the office," I pointed out. "Enough for all of us to have our own, and for keeping separate pencils and pens and Magic Markers and Crayons and paint brushes." I told them not to mix them up and not to leave broken pencils without points, particularly when a sharpener was conveniently affixed to the garage wall. Above all, they were not to touch my two Santa Anita commemorative mugs from the Oak Tree meets of 1988 and 1989 in which I stored my best writing implements.

They all seemed cowed. Even Madeleine, the budding businesswoman for whom the message was mainly meant.

Hah! Unwittingly, I had really let the labeling genie out of the bottle. The next day I found a chartreuse label reading "Dad" across the bay chest of my favorite gelding, John Henry, and on the other beer stein another "Dad" blotting out the likeness of Jockey Chris McCarron. It didn't stop there. Labels had blossomed everywhere, including hand-crafted numerals affixed with Scotch tape to the doors of every room in the house. Apparently, her enthusiasm for labeling had spilled over into her career search, and we'd all become unknowing players in a Motel Owner's fantasy.

Careers in Progress

"Looks like we're in Room 5," I remarked to my wife. "I think it's the bridal suite." I was tempted to pen a note for the concierge asking that Room 5 get a good cleaning and a sheet change. But I thought better of it. No sense encouraging any further unwarranted searches of my dresser drawers and clothes closet.

The next morning I ambled to the kitchen to prepare breakfast and pack lunches for school. Secured to the range hood by magnets were little pre-printed pieces of pulp paper with orders in a familiar hand:

pancakes

scramble eggs

1 cinamon toast

1 locks on toast

tea

dipping eggs

regular toast

jam toast

milk

In two days' time I'd been reduced from resident to transient, and demoted from family chef to fry cook.

I had no objection to my daughter getting an early start on her career plans. In fact, I admired her for it. So there really was only one thing to do. Go forward immediately with the long-discussed room addition, a new study off an expanded living room. She could have the whole house as a bed-and-breakfast if she wanted, with maid and janitorial service provided, I hoped. So long as she didn't expect me to be the short-order cook…and I had a writing room all to my very own.

Memoirs of a Geezer Dad

Lately, and perhaps just in time, action on the fantasy front has slowed.

With the onset of her teenage years, oldest daughter Molly has gone increasingly inside. Reserved, cerebral, and risk-averse, she defines well the word bookish, has straight As in her first three years of high school, and is already shopping for a university to match her scholarly interests. I feel safe predicting for her a future in academia.

Madeleine also seems to have settled on a profession, though I remain more than skeptical. Some months back she informed me with her customary determination that she intended to be a pathologist.

"Why do you want to cut open dead people?" I asked, thinking perhaps she didn't know the job description, and savvy enough not to tell her I thought spending her working day with cadavers was a ghoulish idea.

She was ready for me. "Because doctors hurt people when they are alive. You can't hurt them when they're dead."

True, but...I suggested that instead of a pathologist, she might want to become a veterinarian because she absolutely adores animals and has a real way with them.

No dice, for the same softhearted reason—she didn't want to hurt any living animal. And I suppose there are no animal pathologists. Anyway, I wrote off her job choice as temporary, one she would soon abandon when she found out how much math—a subject she claims to hate—was required.

Wrong again. Within the past month I eavesdropped on her and her brother Franz in the car as they discussed their futures. My ears perked up when I heard her say, "I'm not going to get married, and I'm going to have a house full of pets."

"But what are you going to *do?*" Franz asked, an open-ended question to be sure.

"I'm going to be a pathologist."

Franz did not know the word. "What do they do?"

"They cut open dead people to find out what killed them."

"Ugh!" Franz said. "Why would you want to do that?"

"Because if you're a surgeon and you make a mistake you kill the person. If you're a pathologist, they're already dead."

Same sound reasoning as before. Franz, though, apparently couldn't deal with the idea head-on, so he launched into a discussion of his own future. "I'll probably be a millionaire," he said with an air of resignation.

"Why?" Maddy asked, clearly a doubter.

"Because I'll be a Major League baseball player, and they get about nine million a year."

This was too much even for the supportive geezer, who does everything he can to encourage his children. "Maybe you should think of a back-up career, just in case," I interrupted. "You've always liked the sciences."

Franz didn't miss a beat: "I know. After I'm retired from baseball, I'm going to be a paleontologist."

That would probably be the first such career change—from fastballs to fossils—on record. But what could I say other than "Go for it!" This was, after all, the boy who at age six went around the house singing to himself, "Don't want to work, not gonna work, never gonna work." The melody overheard by the rest of us was no big thing, but the words reeked of a conviction borne out in every family work project since, from which he pulled a vanishing act worthy of Harry Houdini.

I have good reason to believe his sloth is not terminal. Give him the chance to play, and he does so virtually around the clock, with great gusto. It's as though he's following the classroom advice I used to give young college men and women when they fretted over their future careers. "The secret to life," I would tell them, "is to make work play. And vice versa."

Memoirs of a Geezer Dad

Now if Franz, my final hostage to fortune, my little boy of such potential, the offspring I'll probably never know as an adult, one of the three very reasons for this book being written, can only make play work. And vice versa.

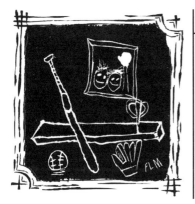

Chapter 10

The Boy
and Geezer
of Summer

PART FROM A sense of humor (the *sine qua non* for survival in this particular universe), for me the most amazing quality of humans is their power to fantasize. The ability to transcend our mere selves through the power of imagination—leave dull and undistinguished lives to become heroes and heroines in our nourishing make-believe worlds.

I am reminded of this almost daily by my young son who walks around with a bat or football or basketball in hand, all the while broadcasting in shrill and muffled narrative his imaginary doings in the wonderful world of sports. I try not to eavesdrop. But every now and then I will catch a name—Kobe Bryant, John Elway, or Sammy Sosa—in the private radiocast. More often, though, I hear the broadcaster's own name, Franz, who doubles as a contender against the best, in whatever sport.

At times I've been tempted to ask him to turn up the volume, so I can share the excitement. But I resist. My policy is to not intrude, lest I lessen his mastery of his private universe and do lasting damage. This pays off in the occasional news bulletin he sends my way, such as "I'm catching Roberto Alomar for the batting crown."

"I'm pulling for you. Just keep your swing level," I say, trying to reinforce good habits, even when taken to his imaginary world.

Yes, it takes a dreamer to know one. Or to encourage one. And I see evidence I am not alone. Fathers who live vicariously

101

Memoirs of a Geezer Dad

through the athletic deeds of their sons or daughters catch a lot of flack these days. Mostly deserved. Usually it's connected with some boorish behavior from the sidelines or grandstand directed against coaches or referees. While I don't count myself among the boors, I readily confess to basking in the early athletic career of Franz. How could I not when it so outshines my own?

Franz is, as they say, a natural. Rangy and muscular, his quickness, strength, and grace complement neatly his instinctive knowledge of each game's fine points of strategy. Moreover, he brings these gifts to virtually every sport he plays. His first try at soccer revealed a defensive tiger of a middle fielder who could also score when called upon; the second year he earned the nickname "horse" while averaging 1.5 goals a game. When I was young under the California sun that Old World game was not even an option.

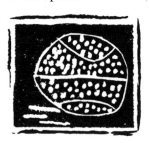

Introduced to basketball at age seven, he led his toothless 2–6 Panthers in scoring, rebounding, and steals, excelling in one-on-one situations where his great tactical speed led to breakaway lay-ups. My roundball career was mostly spent riding the pine, a lead-footed garbage forward brought in when the game was pretty much settled or a starter had fouled out.

It was after his overmatched Panthers got thrashed 80–12 in a game (he was high-point boy, with 12) that I asked him a question that had been building in my mind.

The Boy and Geezer of Summer

"Son, do you ever feel nervous in a game?"

He looked at me strangely, as though his authority on all things bright and beautiful had lost his marbles.

"I mean, do you ever get butterflies in your belly...maybe before a game?"

"Dad!" he remonstrated. "It's *fun*."

Wow! What a refutation. I guess it must be so, if it comes that easily. I resolved then and there that I would continue to be nervous for him, from the grandstand, vicariously. It's the least I can do.

Baseball remains his first love, as it was mine and my father's before me. My father was a fine left-handed, line-drive-hitting first baseman. I showed some promise as a pitcher before the Korean War pretty much nipped any professional prospects in the bud. But Franz—showing it from age eight and after—is in a higher league than either of us. For his coach-pitch team, the rather ordinary 6–8 Rockies, he hit an astonishing .684 and with power (league-leading seven home runs and 24 RBIs); stepping up to the hapless 2 – 15 Mets in the kid-pitch minor league, he lead his team in batting (.413) and pitching ERA (2.87).

The problem? He knows how good he is. And vanity has raised its ugly and highly visible head. Between innings he will seek me out—official scorekeeper camped out behind third base—for a statistical update on his batting average. "Get back with your teammates," I scold aloud, embarrassed for him. (I kept my stats, too, when I played, but secretly, in my head. No need for the world to know I was a lifelong .252 opposite-field banjo-hitter.)

Yes, I firmly believe you should always build your child up, encourage him or her. But can you take the positive approach too far? Foster unreasonable expectations? How do you strike a proper balance?

Memoirs of a Geezer Dad

I have delivered soft sermons to my son on how there is no "I" in the word "team." I paraphrase John Wooden's wise words about playing the best you can and not paying much mind to final scores and who won and who lost and averages and such. (One look at any cemetery's stones tells you that everyone loses in the last inning.)

How little impression my preaching had made on him came after a game in which he drove one deep in the left-center-field alley for a winning three-run homer in the last half-inning. In the general post-game jubilation he accepted in stride what were becoming regular congratulations from his admiring teammates. Initially, I felt reassured. Maybe he had learned to keep his hat size after all.

"Dad," he said in a grave tone on the drive home from the game. "I want to play in the National League."

It took me a few seconds to comprehend what he meant…the grandness of his illusion. He was talking about the National League, as in the *Major League National League!* "Why?" I asked, suspecting I knew the answer.

"Because we know I'm a great pitcher *and* a great hitter. I want to do both, and they don't let pitchers bat in the American League."

"That's true," I said. I then delivered my finest-yet lecture on taking one's time in making life-determining decisions and how our expectations should always stay flexible. There was still high school and college—not to mention the bulk of grammar school—to be got through before a hard decision had to be made.

He listened without comment.

The following Monday when I picked him from school I asked my ritual question: "What did you do today?"

Which got me the ritual answer: "Nothun."

"Well, did you talk to anybody today?"

The Boy and Geezer of Summer

"Yes, I told a girl I hit the winning home run."
"What did she say?"
"Nothun."
I left unsaid the advice he should have heard: "Hey, Dude. Don't bore chicks with baseball. Tell them their hair looks nice and get their phone numbers." On second thought, that could wait…a long time.

Sports is not the only thing that brings my son and me close. But it remains the dominant thing, comfortably ahead of the subject of dinosaurs. His enthusiasm for team sports seems boundless, even as mine wanes with age. For me, watching soccer is even less inviting than playing it. Hockey appeals to folks who like their violence more authentic than the WWF dishes out. Football over time has become a dreary dumb show of oafs and future violent offenders, the particulars of its individual contests interchangeable—particularly at the professional level. Basketball can be exciting, especially if your alma mater makes it to March Madness…yet the games are strangely forgettable—rapid come, rapid go. For me, only the sublime game baseball has staying power, and whether I watch my son play it or we watch a televised game together, I don't have to fake enthusiasm to match his.

I believe that one of my greatest gifts to my son has been feeding his own love of the game, introducing him to the summers of bliss that have mythic status in the American experience. Baseball, it seems to me, is a game of the past and the present, not the future. And in America it unites fathers and sons. For my father and me it was the one constant, our communing ground, limited as it was. Most of the pleasant memories I have of that tall, stern and stoic German involve baseball,

Memoirs of a Geezer Dad

going all the way back to 1938 and my first Major League game in Cleveland's old League Park. That day I embarrassed him by screaming through a lightning storm until the game was called in the early innings, and we were given our precious Depression Days' rain check. Appropriately enough, Roy "Stormy" Weatherly (my early favorite Cleveland Indian) hit a homer that was scratched. That's about all I can remember of the game, besides the park's high walls and the frightening lightning and deafening thunder and my own five-year-old's shame at crying hysterically in public.

Separated by temperament, my father and I used the game to explore our relationship. Even here we could be adversarial. In the early 1940s I touted my favorite member of the Tribe, Jeff Heath, stationed in left field where we usually sat at Cleveland Municipal Stadium, as the American League's best hitter. He countered with his idol, Ted Williams, whom he claimed was the greatest hitter ever and advised me to model myself after him. He was right, and I was wrong not to model myself after the Splendid Splinter (though I console myself with the knowledge that no one else has either).

At a picnic in about 1941, when I tried vainly to get the beer-swilling adults to break from their gabfest for a baseball game, my unusually talkative father took me aside and said he understood my love of the game. He loved it, too, and my very unplanned coming scotched his tryout with the Chicago White Sox. Instead, he had to seek hard-to-come-by and unglamorous work as a machinist with the New York Central Railroad.

What he innocently thought was a shared secret that would lead to intimacy instead planted the seed of guilt in my receptive mind. Somehow, I've never shaken the vague blame for him failing to realize his life's dream.... I had thwarted his career by my very being.

106

The Boy and Geezer of Summer

Baseball was the credo I pushed on the three sons of my first family, and I still freshly recall in detail coaching my twin eleven-year-olds Kurt and Karl to the 1978 San Fernando Valley's Little League championship game, which we lost 9–8 in the bottom of the ninth on my poor base-running call from the first-base coaching box. (If only I had replaced the limping Andy Eckoff on the basepaths before my son Kurt caught up with him on third while legging out his aborted triple.)

I waited until Franz (whose first word was "ball") was four months shy of reaching four years before taking him to his first Major League baseball game, a May match between the California Angels and the Cleveland Indians. Would he fret as kids do, get bored, misbehave in order to force an early departure? Not at all. "The Indians are having a meeting," he said early to describe a mound conference. And even though the game was a tight 1–1 pitching duel into the ninth inning—before fireballer Troy Percival gave up three monster home-run blasts to Albert Belle, Sandy Alomar, and Jim Thome—Franz sat patiently, absorbing more than I thought. On the drive home he correctly reported that "the Indians hit three homeruns and the Angels had one." *Awesome!*

Let me admit that encouraging my last boy to play baseball brought with it obligations I've met rather poorly. It's not enough to tout the glorious game unbound by time, with its intervals of frozen moments and fluid moves borrowed from chess and ballet and played on the pastures of heaven. Dads are supposed to teach their sons to throw, catch, hit…until more knowledgeable (or in my case, more physically able) coaches can take over.

Memoirs of a Geezer Dad

I did well enough at first, playing catch with him on our postage-stamp-sized front lawn. Then I pitched him whiffleballs, and he pitched them to me in what became hotly contested, improvised games I had to be careful not to always win. Arguments arose, and we took ad hoc action to continually add to a growing compendium of ground rules. But by the Tee Ball stage my gout, arthritis, or bursitis was acting up so often that I spent three days on the disabled list for every game on the field with my favorite Tee-Baller.

Feeling guilty, I tried coaxing him inside to watch games on television. As tube tubers together, we could discuss and learn the multitudinous fine points of baseball strategy from a comfortable couch. After all, among sports, baseball was the ultimate head game. Its mental side was just as important as the physical...maybe more so.

Franz bought into my ploy for quite some time. But he absorbed the game's complexities so quickly—all the subtle moves and countermoves, short-run tactics, and long-range strategies—that I soon realized I was in the presence of a six-year-old reincarnation of Whitey Herzog.

The epiphany came on one spring afternoon while we were tube-watching Oakland and Cleveland play, and Indian left fielder Will Cordero got hit on the hand. He had to leave the game, and Cleveland manager Mike Hargrove sent Richie Sexson in to play left field for him.

"Hargrove made a mistake," muttered my son.

"How's that?" I asked, realizing a second later that he was absolutely right.

"Because he should have moved Justice from DH to left and used Sexon as DH. Justice is a much better fielder than Sexson."

Right on! Management in Cleveland must have shared

The Boy and Geezer of Summer

his analysis because in a matter of months Hargrove got his walking papers.

Clearly a holder of credentials to be a Major League manager if he doesn't make the Show as a player, Franz's interest in our skull sessions soon tapered off. This old spud could still occasionally lure him into sharing the La-Z-Boy—particularly if one of his favorite teams (the Dodgers or the Rockies, namesakes of his own teams) were playing. But it wasn't long before the action on the tube incited him. I would look away when he started swinging his plastic bat or a stick or an empty gift wrap tube and he slammed a whiffleball, sponge, or rolled sock around the living room in violation of house rules. Sometimes I even consented to pitching duty, lobbing a sock or Nerfball toward his wicked swings, but usually I just tried to watch the televised game. He couldn't help acting out what we were watching, catching tosses into his glove while falling, or accidentally slamming his bat against the coffee table—all the while broadcasting the action in a muted-but-excited, high-pitched boy's voice that meant to mimic the parables of Vin Scully. All too soon, though, he wearied of the confinement and headed outside to find a neighbor kid to play with. My aching back would sigh with relief when the door slammed.

One day, at the start of a recent season when apparently no neighborhood boy was available, he sought me out at my place before the 18-inch Sony.

"Dad, throw me some out front."

"I can't, son," I pled with my customary guilt. "My shoulder's shredded."

"Please, Dad. The season's starting, and I need the hitting practice."

"Hey! Why not watch a game with me on the telly? Your Dodgers are playing."

Memoirs of a Geezer Dad

"I've got a better idea," he said, face brightening. He left and returned in seconds with a plastic bat and a rolled-up pair of socks. "Just toss me some from the chair so I can work on my swing."

"You know Mom doesn't allow that in the living room anymore," I reminded him.

"Mom isn't here."

True. Out shopping, no surprise. Took his sisters—future shoppers in training—with her. That eliminated any snitches.

And so the lazy geezer reclining in the La-Z-Boy started lobbing across his body a rolled-up pair of socks that Franz slashed around the living room. Luckily, the cat and dog had sought cover, and the furniture is durable...or disposable. (Furnishing your home in Goodwill Modern does offer a few advantages.) Besides, whatever gets broken now can be replaced from that multi-year, multi-million-dollar contract in the future when, if all goes well, I'll be looking down on Franz's Major League career from horsehide heaven.

There I go again. That's the kind of dangerous, unrealistic fantasizing that makes boors of fathers and ruins their sons, and I condemn myself and others for putting so much pressure on children to make it in professional sports. Actually, I'd settle for a college baseball scholarship for the kid.

Mea culpa again for the narrow, selfish thinking. Wrongheaded as well. Yes, athletics may bind some fathers and sons, yet still set them up for the harsh reality that professional athletes are few, while the near-misses and also-rans are legion. Of course, there are many other fathers for whom athletics play no part at all in the father-son relationship. Not to mention those boys whose fathers neglect them entirely or those with no fathers at all.

Lurking behind the myriad real-life links of fathers and sons is the larger question, how do you turn boys into men?

The Boy and Geezer of Summer

Specifically, how do you preserve—even nourish—the sensitivity of a young boy who will find it valuable in future intimate relations with loved ones and, as important, open him to the balm of beauty and the truth of art? How do you maximize the making of the whole man, what was once quaintly known as a gentleman, a true gentleman, with the word shorn of elitist trappings and condescension, a man who treated his alleged inferiors and his alleged superiors as he did his peers, with respect and generosity? The autonomous man? The modest man whose word could be counted on?

What I *don't* mean are the guys you see depicted in beer commercials or at ringside in WWF matches, or hear on sport-radio call-in shows. Not the marks of marketers and media hustlers always looking for consumers and followers.

In my experience, girls have an easier time growing up. They have a stronger sense of self and what's expected of them; they handle their feelings better. Boys trying to be men have a much harder time of it as the need for hunters and warriors diminishes with the creation of each new silicon chip.

I suppose I'm just talking out loud about my major worry as a geezer father raising a young and hypersensitive son. Franz may be athletic, but he is also thoughtful, charitable, gentle, non-combative. While it's a personal joy to live with such a boy, those same qualities have already left him vulnerable outside the home. Let us be true to one another, dads of the world: Sensitivity doesn't help much in the male world out there that's knocked us about. Bury your feelings, we were told. Toughen up, kill or be killed, etc. We may prescribe early karate lessons for our sons, or look away when our adolescents pick up coarse language or experiment with controlled substances. Those are established signposts on the road to manhood, which is just south of macholand.

111

Memoirs of a Geezer Dad

All of which points up both the importance of and the confusion over role models. I believe most boys live to prove themselves to their fathers (or father substitutes). Gain their approval, early and often. Sadly, too many fathers withhold it, as if the act of praising or commending somehow stunts a boy's growth. My father was reluctant to ever praise his three sons directly. But if we were eavesdropping, we sometimes heard him bragging about us to others. Lately I've found myself doing the same thing, brought to my attention by my son who picks up every plaudit, even when he's seemingly not listening. So in an exercise I call "reversing the sins of the father," I force myself to compliment all my children face to face when they do something noteworthy.

Of course, the definition of a "sin" can change over time. I found my father guilty of such a sin one watershed day when I was nine. Though a reluctant combatant always, I suddenly found myself in an all-out fist fight on my front lawn with the neighbor boy Robert. I was doing well enough, had him down and was on top of him, when his eight-year-old brother David whacked me from behind and knocked me off. Together they pounded me pretty well before my father appeared. He wasted some seconds watching the lopsided combat before tardily pulling them both off me. He showed me no emotion at all and offered no comforting words as I went into the house blubbering about the injustice done me.

For a time I held a grudge against my father for letting the battle continue. For not intervening promptly and marching next door to settle scores with the parents of Robert and David. I saw his conduct consistent with his view of me as "emotional" (a euphemism for "sissy-in-training"), having heard him when he was in his cups with friends refer to me as "Jeannette's boy." Mama's boy. Two more sons would follow me, more like him in manly temperament.

The Boy and Geezer of Summer

But later in life I modified my resentment. In his way, my father was merely preparing me for life and the competitive and unforgiving society of young males with their hormones at flood tide. The lesson was driven home in my second day of boot camp, at Lackland Air Force Base back in September of 1951, when Corporal Mount faced our flight of raw recruits in formation and bellowed, "You play ball with me...[pause]...and I'll shove the bat up your ass!" It took a few moments before the meaning of the surprise punchline sank in. We could toady and suck-up and do what we were told, and we'd still be in for some heavy abuse. Which, of course, we were. The bottom line of all that was "toughen up," perhaps encapsulated best in the contemporary bumper sticker, "No Whining."

I survived. Virtually all of us did. Had to. But hardened to someone no longer a boy. I knew it from the forlorn way my mother looked at me when I came home on my first leave, a look that said, "I have lost the son I knew." As indeed she had. The cord was clipped. The new distance, sadly, endured.

Franz will probably never undergo military basic training to harden him—or break him. So how will his mettle be tested? By people and events I'll likely never know. I've listened with interest lately to sports heroes begging off role-model duty. In a way, I understand why if I don't actually applaud what I see as their selfishness. They don't want any more external obligations cramping their style...curtailing their conduct.

But fathers can't beg off so easily. Biology, with an assist from society, casts us as role models to our children. And others judge how well we perform. Which leads me to go back and examine my own performance the first time around, when I was both vigorous and self-absorbed and invoked the slightly specious "do-as-I-say, not-as-I-do" method of child rearing. Though I've checked with my three grown sons, and they give me fairly high marks for preparing them for manhood, I was a

Memoirs of a Geezer Dad

party to a messy divorce that scrambled their lives when they were 11 and 12 years old. In giving them a traditional masculine model, I did all right. Regrettably, I did so in part by living the advertisers' version, with harmful consequences to my sons and me. I smoked for 27 years…until I finally mustered the will to overcome the addiction. They smoked; two of them quit in their twenties, but one continues on into his late-thirties. I drank, sometimes to excess, until the time I had a second family and realized I was unlikely to see them enter high school unless I gave up suds and juniper juice. I stopped. My sons indulged early, then relaxed back into moderation. Little harm, minor foul…I hope.

On the positive side of the ledger, I spent seasons coaching them in baseball and basketball, the stuff still of bonding memories that often surface at extended family reunions. I also watched back then a lot of televised sports, but only one of the three bought into that inexpensive waste of time.

In my second round of parenting I've become much more

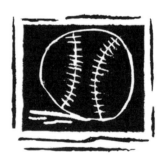

involved in my children's lives. My motto: Less life to live; more care to give. I hope my immersion will help guide them in the right way and leave more memories of me that stick in their minds…and stick in mine as sustenance for my remaining days.

The Boy and Geezer of Summer

Most poignant for me in recent years was the August day I accompanied Franz, my sixth and last child, on his first day of school. Actually, it was a summer day camp preview of what his Catholic kindergarten would be like the coming month—introduction day, as it were:

Even as I help him put on the logoed shirt, emblazoned "Sonshine Summer," that will be his summer uniform, I notice my tall, blond, baseball-loving five-year-old is a scared raw rookie in a new league. He balks at donning the blue lei he is supposed to wear to the first day's gathering on the school playing field.

"The other kids will be wearing their leis," I tell him, disgusted with myself for playing the peer-pressure card so early.

He reluctantly slips it on. But he also pulls on his Dodger cap, a defensive gesture, I think, one that reassures him as to his identity. He isn't saying much. Isn't saying anything at all.

At the field gathering, two competent girls in their teens direct us to the groups assembling under identifying pole-borne placards. I find "K-3," Franz's new and temporary group identity and stand there with six mothers and one other father. I note that we serve as leaning posts for shrinking children who clearly would prefer to be elsewhere.

Katie, a smiling counselor in her early twenties, approaches us with name badges and asks Franz, "What is your name?"

His chin falls to his chest; his mouth clamps shut.

"He's Franz," I say.

"Oh yes. I've got yours here. Where should I pin it?"

Head still downcast, the boy points to the area of his navel, where Katie obligingly pins it.

As Katie moves on to other pinning duties, Franz

stealthily slips off his lei and hands it to me. I look around. Sure enough, only two other kids are wearing their leis. Next I'm furtively handed the Dodger hat. No one else is true blue. Peer pressures, I learn, operate under their own natural laws, not as I would apply them.

About now with my first family I would have vamoosed. Clapped all three boys heartily on the back, given them a "go-get-'em" shout of encouragement, and then been on my way to the working world where career and accomplishment, such as they were, awaited me. But this day I have the mind and luxury to linger.

Franz's fear is growing. For support, I rub his slumping shoulders and whisper in his ear, as though it were a fact, "You're going to have a great time."

The counselors have now gathered all the children into a great circle. One self-assured young woman then leads the assembled in an opening prayer. Though an eternal doubter, I nevertheless make the sign of the cross, in reflexive respect for tradition and in deference to the faithfulwho surround me. Then the same young woman, with obvious leadership qualities, proposes that we sing ensemble that cloying staple of Christian campfires everywhere, "Kumbaya."

She leads us in fine voice. Very few of the assembled follow at first. That builds to a majority. I try to join, but several swelling lumps push the words back into my bronchial tree.

Foolish, mawkish me? Yes, but I don't think it's the song. It's the sight of my son, who has shrunk back to lean hard against me, head still down, lips compressed. I am saddened at this suggestion that he is my son, shy as I was shy, seeking the fringe of the crowd, possibly destined for the limiting loneliness that comes with feeling you don't belong.

After another joyous song of belief, all the children are

called to join one hand-holding circle. I have to push him forward to join it. General announcements are made, then groups are reformed, and each is led off to a classroom to a buoyant chorus of young women promising fun and more inside.

I see my son's head raise a little. He is the tallest child in his group. Handsome, too, in this father's wet eye.

The lumps remain in my throat as I turn away and hope that his reticence—that handicap I likely gave him with my genes—will prove only a temporary condition, perhaps brought on by the occasion, typical of the first-day-of-school syndrome. After a couple days or maybe a week, he'll probably adjust and actually be the solid cement for a group of timid five-year-olds going through a hard rite of passage we demand of them in the complex lives we nowadays live.

But then again, there will be many, many other occasions and rites to come. Will the shyness return, time and again? Will he find the same costly relief I ultimately found, in alcohol? I sure hope not. But isn't that weakness genetically transmitted? Then what or whom will he lean on?

I pray I can be his teary-eyed pillar and protector for decades to come.

Are you listening, Lord?

Geezer fathers and grandfathers alike are allowed to lapse into bourgeois sentimentality on first days of school. Ditto on those infrequent evenings when the boy still chooses to sit in the lap of the lazy geezer in the La-Z-Boy and watch with me the TV tuned to a ballgame or a Nova show on dinosaurs. Down he plops. Ouch!

Memoirs of a Geezer Dad

Heir to paternal genes that assure a height of between 6' 2" and 6' 6" when fully grown, and razor-edged bones that won't add flesh until the distant side of 30, he's already well beyond lap size. His elbows carve new holes in my tired old flesh. I wince and shift my weight and muffle all cries of pain, because I don't want him to feel unwelcome while grinding down my hip bone which, if I'm lucky, will be plastic in a few years.

When the pain becomes too much, I'll excuse myself on the pretext of a bathroom run or a glass of water, rise and shake out my joints and fluff out my liver. But I always go back for more. I don't want to lose physical contact with my last child. I already know it will come soon enough. And when he does grow too old to sit in Dad's lap, I will look back with deepest regrets at having lost that touch.

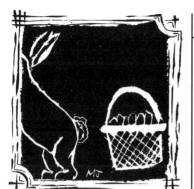

Chapter 11

Myths
and
Their Undoing

THE TOOTH FAIRY, the Easter Bunny, and Santa Claus are old acquaintances, not necessarily my friends. This is my third go-round with them. First time it was as a receiving believer in an era of low expectations, the second and third times as the reluctant power and pocketbook behind the myths we use to soften life for our children and point them in the direction of faith. (Even as we undermine it with the bogus trio, I might observe.)

I can't say I'm altogether comfortable in the role. And that is probably why I'm rather inept in performing my part in the time-worn rituals. With my first family I went along because it was the thing to do. The second time I debated with myself, briefly, to be sure, whether the clean cold honesty of the plain and simple truth wasn't preferable to furthering illusions that cost money and, later, trust. Yes, yes, I know the good vibrations these canards send throughout the family, and that's probably why they occupy their hallowed places in our lives.

The Tooth Fairy is my least favorite of the trinity. A skeptic early, I cast out belief in him or her or it years before the Easter Bunny and Santa Claus got the cognitive heave-ho. That may explain my failure to remember details of the deception I had been through five previous times before six-year-old Franz approached me on what his worried face told me was an urgent matter.

Memoirs of a Geezer Dad

"I think I'm going to lose my first tooth today," he said, jiggling a lower incisor between thumb and forefinger. "It's halfway sealed out of my gums."

Indeed it was. No sooner had the news circulated through the household than my tradition-adoring wife set in motion the practiced protocol. She talked up the event, then got out the little pillow with the little pocket sewn for this very rite by his Aunt Maggie. My main responsibility was to come up with three dollar bills and put them into the little pocket on the little pillow that rested near his sleeping head.

Three dollars? "Isn't that a bit much?" I asked my wife, who has special knowledge of all the fine points of domestic rituals. (There was a Tooth Fairy practicing in Cleveland, Ohio, when I lost my first tooth, but the big news then was Hitler's invasion of Poland, not the nickel left under my pillow.)

"No, it's the going rate for a first tooth," she said. "It's gone up since you were a boy."

For sure. Inflation happens. What hadn't suffered its ravages over 60 years? Except, of course, my prospects.

The tooth promptly lost its hold in the gums. Something seemed to be bothering my young son, though. "What's wrong?" I asked.

"It's very small," Franz said.

I inspected the tooth. It was indeed very small, easily overlooked by a Tooth Fairy on a tight tooth-buying schedule.

Nine-year-old Madeleine—still a believer herself and a stickler like Mom for tradition—quickly solved our problem. She Magic-Markered a letter-sized white envelope in bold blue letters the TF couldn't miss:

WARNING: Franz's tooth very small.

Franz seemed reassured when he went to sleep. I waited until midnight before I slipped into his room to deftly tuck the three bills into the little pocket on the little pillow.

"Done," I said in the hall to my waiting wife.

"Where's the tooth?"

"Tooth?"

"Yes, your son's first tooth that's in the white envelope under the pillow!" she said in consternation.

Duh.

I returned and just as deftly snaked the envelope out from under the sleeping boy's head. Done to perfection.

Franz said nothing when he awoke the next morning. I got nervous. He couldn't have forgotten to look for his take.

"Well, did the Tooth Fairy come?" I asked.

"Yeah," he said, with some obvious disappointment.

"What did you get?"

"Three dollars."

"Wow! You don't seem very happy?"

"Mark got five dollars for his."

I was stunned and doubly resentful of the whole Tooth Fairy scam. Mark, a schoolmate of his, was, if anything, of a lower socioeconomic station. What if Franz shared with his mates news of his economic shortfall? Inquiring minds might see behind Franz's stingy Tooth Fairy the specter of "old penny-pinching Dad," as the three sons of my first family liked to refer to me. (Maybe Franz himself would echo those words one day.) I, too, was disappointed.

Memoirs of a Geezer Dad

The next day he came at me with one of his subtly probing questions: "What happens with the skin that goes over the molar when you get that one?"

I was momentarily baffled and asked him to repeat the question, which he did, adding "you know, the skin that covers the tooth. Does it come out?"

"The skin that covers the tooth?" I decided to just wing it. "Well, that just becomes a flap that heals in your mouth, like, you know, when you get a cut finger and a scab forms."

He looked crestfallen.

"What's wrong?"

"The Tooth Fairy can't give money for that, then?"

"No, I'm afraid not."

"I was hoping she might give more for that."

What ingratitude! What inflated expectations! He should fare well in the new global economy with an attitude like that.

I thought of snuffing the myth right there and then. Cast the Tooth Fairy into the bright light of truth and be rid forever of the non-existent nuisance.

No, I couldn't. Age has brought me a smattering of wisdom. You don't dash beliefs and rites that sustain others…unless you have something darn good and effective to put in their places. And I don't.

"Look on the bright side," I said with feigned heartiness to my son. "You've got a lot more teeth to lose." (When the Tooth Fairy cometh, he, she, or it cometh again and again and again.)

The long-awaited first return, or dreaded return, depending on who you were, came three-and-a-half months later. Actually, it came and went.

"Tomorrow I'm going to get some money," Franz announced to me as I drove him to school after a morning of hectic preparation.

Myths and Their Undoing

"Really? From whom?"

"The Tooth Fairy. She forgot to come last night."

Oh no! I forgot! After several self-reminders during the day and a final one from my wife before she retired, I forgot! The little guy had trustingly put his little tooth into the little pocket sewn on the little pillow—no white envelope this time—and came up with…a tooth. No bucks. Shame on me!

"She didn't come?" I asked rhetorically and lamely.

"That's okay. She's going to bring me four dollars tonight."

Four dollars! He was charging a 33% late-payment penalty! That's usurious, unfair. Or was the little guy a lot more aware than he seemed and was just working a scam, pretending faith for a suitable reward?

He spoke and I immediately felt more guilt for my cynical suspicions. "Is there more than one Tooth Fairy, Dad?"

"Probably so, son."

"Why?"

"Because there are billions of children in the world losing teeth, and she can't be everywhere." To break off contact, I walked down the hall and waded into his room to see if he had left out the pillow for the cash deposit. He had, tooth enclosed. But he had also left his room a mess, with wall-to-wall toys obstructing access.

"No wonder the Tooth Fairy didn't come," I said, looking for an alibi wherever it might be found. "Who could even get into this room with all these toys blocking the way?"

"Dad," he countered with sudden disgust. "The Tooth Fairy can fly."

I had forgotten that.

That evening, after I carried him to bed from the living room where he'd fallen asleep watching a baseball game, I re-waded through the room to the little pillow on his bed. I counted out one, two, *three* dollar bills…and slipped them into the

Memoirs of a Geezer Dad

little pocket. I left feeling relieved—and pleased. I had held the line.

"Where's the tooth?" my wife asked me in the hall.

Sheepishly, I returned to the pillow and fished out from under the folded bills a tiny incisor with a red-brown spot where the root had been. The tooth was no larger than the first. I gave it to my wife who immediately choked up with excess emotion.

"It's so small," she whispered. "Our little boy is growing up so quickly. I'll put this with the other one."

I averted my face, refusing to share her mawkish feelings over the fleetness of time and the brevity of life. I had just stood shoulder to shoulder with Alan Greenspan as another hard-nosed enemy of inflation.

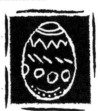

With the Easter Bunny, I get along. His (her?) impact on the household is minimal, for what reason I'm not exactly sure. Maybe it's because my wife takes care of all the details, and I don't have to lift a finger. Maybe it's because our pagan visitor brings only candy and eggs, exacts no cash on the barrel-head, doesn't traffic in toys that are bought and bought and over-bought. By my happy reckoning, the cost of candy and eggs is 2.7% (you can check it out) of what Saint Nick nicks us for. I should also mention that I get salvage rights to any partially eaten chocolate eggs left adhering to the upholstery, which always amounts to too much of a good thing for my touchy stomach.

In checking my journal notes to confirm that in our home

the Easter Bunny is a relatively neglected presence, lacking the eclat of the Tooth Fairy and Santa, I find only a few entries on the subject.

One is from my daughter Madeleine when she was six, and Easter was around the corner.

"Are you allergic to rabbits?" she asked me.

"I don't know. Why do you ask?"

"Because you're allergic to cats."

"Rabbits are not cats."

"The Easter Bunny will probably leave some fluff when he comes," she explained.

I was truly thankful for the heads-up.

My son, again at age six, prompted the second entry.

"The Easter Bunny sure is intelligent," he informed me, out of the blue. (Or would it be the pink?)

"Why do you say that?"

"He knew just what I wanted."

"What was that?" I wondered aloud, knowing it wasn't the dozen uneaten yellow sugar-coated chicks I'd just thrown in the garbage.

"A basketball."

"A basketball?"

"Yes, just what I wanted."

I didn't quarrel with the choice, just that the Easter Bunny (who wasn't any brighter than the Tooth Fairy, as far as I was concerned) was encroaching on Santa's turf. And that spelled an even greater family budget deficit—a matter to be discussed with the wife.

For me Christmas is the season to be wary. It's when budgets burst, and Franz picks up again the grilling of his old man

Memoirs of a Geezer Dad

on a recurring subject—the existence of Santa Claus.

Our Christmas season actually begins the first week of December. That's the deadline for donating toys to Corazon, our local church charity that sends collected items to children in Mexico. Delivery day is preceded by a three-day ritual at our house in which boxes, bags, and piles of toys cluttering the garage are brought in and sorted into givers and keepers.

Ever the optimist, I hope annually for an outburst of Christian charity and that the give-away pile wins in a toy-slide. That would give me clear sailing to clean the garage before Santa comes and dumps more impedimenta in the house, and the garage again fills with the overflow.

Alas! Not to be this most recent year...again. The original six huge, bulging Hefty bags of charitable candidates get gone through and subtracted from until reduced to a flabby three and a half. The pack-rat gene wins again. (And it's not from any chromosome of mine, either!) Well, I console myself with the Monty Python guys' advice to look on the bright side of life—at least I won't have to clean the garage for another year.

The delivery of the toys to Corazon ushers in Act Two of our Christmas Pageant: The preparation of the "want" lists via letters to Santa. Time for me to submerge my Scroogean impulses and guard against verbal blunders that would kill the spirit of Christmas present. As for Christmas presents, my wife catches the spirit of the season in three weeks of concentrated fury, assaulting the malls trebly armed with cash, plastic, and checkbook. (I confine my shopping to a two-hour window on the evening of December 23, when you can really find some terrific mark-downs on the uncluttered bins and shelves.)

Most of the rest of the Yuletide, I am busy costarring with my son in Act III of an ongoing courtroom drama that might be called "Santa on Trial." Now in its third year, I appear for the defense of the jolly old fraud, while Franz plays the part of ambivalent plaintiff, torn between the need to believe in this generous bringer of toys and his own relentless skepticism rooted in the need to know.

Franz, age 6: "Is Santa real?"

Dad, nimble in a crisis moment: "Where do you think all those presents come from?"

Franz: "Dad, where does Santa get his toys?"

Dad: "From his elves at the North Pole, I guess. That's what they say, anyway." (That's my favorite double-hedge; I put all fanciful notions in the mouths and minds of others, unwilling to be a party to such deceptions and offend my skeptic's conscience.)

Franz: "Is there a South Pole, too?"

Dad: "Yes, there is…but it's imaginary, you know. It's not a real pole."

Franz: "It doesn't stick up?"

Dad: "No, it's just an imaginary place where the earth ends." (Not a very good explanation.) "It's a mathematical point on the top of an oblate sphere." (He's supposed to understand that? I'm not certain I do. And the "top"? Einstein wouldn't approve of that description of his universe. How about a small-sized planet orbiting a medium-sized star removed from the center of the Milky Way Galaxy, in which all directions are relative and must be arbitrarily assigned from imagined fixed points. And how could I begin to explain all that when I got a D in high school physics, let alone field questions that I have never heard before?)

Franz: "Dad?"

Memoirs of a Geezer Dad

Dad: "Yes."

Franz: "Do Santa's elves work most all the year?"

Dad: "That would make sense, given all the kids in the world."

Franz: "Dad?"

Dad: "Yes?"

Franz: "How do elves make Nintendos?"

Dad: "You ask all the hard questions, don't you? I really don't know."

Franz hesitates a moment before flashing a dismissive look and walking off. I have failed him. But I take consolation that not even Einstein or Planck could have answered the last one.

The following Saturday I took Franz to "Le Grand Mal" (aka South Coast Plaza) to see Santa, thinking it might harden his belief with that tried-and-true bait and switch. Franz seemed nervous.

"What's wrong?" I asked him, noticing he was hesitant to get in the line of 20 or so kids waiting to sit in Santa's lap.

"I don't know what to say."

"Just tell him what you want."

He looked unconvinced. Increasingly, he retreated into his shy mope mode as the line of tots forced him forward toward Santa, who sat on a slightly raised platform and patiently listened to the wants of each mall child before sending him or her down a slide back to a parent. The guy in the loose-fitting red suit seemed, to me at least, sapped of his jollity. Long, hard day, no doubt.

When Franz's time in Santa's brief embrace came, my son sagged inward into a limp bag of bones and kept his lips sealed, before being sent down the slide.

"Why didn't you say anything to him?" I asked.

"I was too shy," he confessed.

Myths and Their Undoing

Apparently his belief in Santa was sustained by the visit even as his confidence in his own abilities was not. He enlisted his older sister to write his Xmas list for him, which he decided to shorten to just one item—a Nintendo 64; he didn't want Saint Nick bringing lesser gifts and overlooking the top priority Nintendo. A couple of days later he added a game as well, figuring the addition wouldn't unduly tax the old fraud's dubious memory.

At least belief was intact...until his seventh Christmas.

Franz, age 7. Weeks before Santa's scheduled coming, the questing questioner returns for further cross-examination.

Franz: "Dad, do you believe in Santa Claus?"

Dad: "Do you?" (I just can't tell direct lies.)

Franz: "Yes."

Dad: "Well, I guess I believe what you believe."

Stony silence, a beetled young brow, and much deep thought before an authoritative announcement.

Franz: "There can be only two persons who give me the presents."

Ouch! He's figured it out. No dodging this time when he asks me the coming question point blank, "It's you and Mom, isn't it?"

Dad: "What two people?" (Always stall is my advice.)

Franz: "Santa Claus or God."

It was my turn to be struck speechless—a good default strategy in any case.

Franz: "And I think I know who it is."

Dad: "Who would that be?" (Asked with relief.)

Franz: "God. God gives them to me."

Dad: "Really? Why do you think so?"

Memoirs of a Geezer Dad

Franz: "Because God made everything. So he made Santa Claus."

Dad: "Good sound reasoning, son." (I always defer to him in matters metaphysical, anyway.)

He started to walk away, then turned and gave me a look—almost detached, rather tutorial—that I had trouble reading. "Dad, did you know that if you don't know the true meaning of Christmas, you can't hear the reindeers' bells or the angel's singing on top of the tree?"

I felt both chastised and wronged. But I nobly bit my tongue.

A few days later Franz caught me laughing at a clever TV ad that showed an out-of-work Santa Claus trying to stay upbeat, a victim with the malls of E-Toy commerce. Franz studied it, then looked to me. I braced myself for a probing line of questioning. But he just stared at me, suspiciously, I thought.

In the hall that night I overheard him questioning his mother in her room.

"Mom, do you believe in Santa Claus?" Consistent with his corroborating instincts. At least two confirming sources. Woodward and Bernstein would applaud this implacable line of inquiry.

"Yes, why do you ask?" (She's a better face-on liar.)

"Some kids don't."

With that pronouncement, I knew Santa would live another year in the hearts of our two youngest children. Which, I have found, is a continued source of general joy in our toy-clogged house.

Belief in the secular trinity reached the breaking point last Christmas, despite my valiant battle to protect the family faith in it. Of course, Molly, the cerebral one, our resident logician, yielded up her own belief in Saint Nick soon after she observed, at age seven, that "it was odd that the Tooth Fairy, Santa Claus, and the Easter Bunny all come at night when we're asleep." But she had the uncommon decency to keep her knowledge to herself, and not spoil the fun for her siblings.

This Christmas past I went to her with the question I felt I already knew the answer to. "Does Madeleine *really* still believe in Santa Claus?"

"Yes, she does," Molly assured me, then paused. "You're going to tell her, aren't you?"

"Tell her there's no Santa Claus? No way!"

"You're going to let her go to high school believing in Santa Claus?" Molly asked, incredulously.

"Well, she'll find out the truth by then...maybe," I added lamely. Maybe not. Madeleine was one of those gifted with faith; one who once memorably confided to her diary in a reverse causal switch, "I love the Easter Bunny, and I believe in him, too." Only the previous Christmas she assured her seven-year-old brother that she would ice some cookies for him to leave by the tree for Santa to snack on after descending the chimney with his bag of swag. On the other hand, some serious cracks in credibility's wall issued from Madeleine that same Christmas Eve. She insisted on leaving by the fireplace, along with the waiting cookie snack and her list of wants, a note that cloaked a challenge: "Most of all I want snow." Tall order. Southern Coastal California where December's daytime local temperature is in the 70s with seldom a cloud puff in sight.

"Santa can't bring snow," my wife told her. "Only God can do that." (She'd obviously been in consultation with Franz on the fine points of theology). Madeleine brushed it off and went to bed expecting miracles.

Memoirs of a Geezer Dad

Time and tide intervened, as they have a habit of doing. Shortly before our last Christmas, Madeleine confronted her mother and me. "There is no Tooth Fairy," she declared defiantly. "You put the money there. There is no Santa Claus either. And there are no magic people."

My wife and I remained silent. We felt her pain, so clear to see in the down-turned frown on her face.

"But I did see the Easter Bunny once," she added, hopefully.

As the accomplished actors we've become, neither my wife nor I smiled, though I was dying for a description of the nimble rabbit who survived the massive icon-smashing.

My wife tried instead to console her on her sudden loss of innocence to the truth that is supposed to make you free. "Don't tell your brother about Santa Claus, please promise me."

Maddy became suddenly animated with the responsibility her new knowledge brought. "Does Molly know?"

"Yes," my wife assured her with a straight face. "But Franz doesn't, and we would like you not to tell him what you've found out."

"I won't," she promised.

"And now that you know, you can help me prepare Franz's stocking."

This appeased the child instantly.

Promise kept? I had reason to wonder—particularly when my favorite cross-examiner cornered me in the La-Z-Boy on Christmas Eve.

"Dad, do you believe in Santa Claus?" the boy asked, with eyes glued to mine for the least sign of deception.

Dad did his practiced dodge: "Do you?"

Franz thought about it. "Yes," he said, falteringly. "Yes…I do."

Dad employed some more slick sophistry: "Well, I believe in you and what you believe."

Promise kept. Faith intact, just barely, and conditionally, I had good reason to believe after talking to Molly. The boy had gone straight to his oldest sister and got her to help him pen a note telling Santa to bring his toys to his bedroom and place them near a foot-high imitation Christmas tree he kept at his bedside. I chalked that up to confirming Santa by sight, the way his sister spotted the Easter Bunny. He also left a cookie for Santa on a plate in the living room next to the family Christmas tree.

The next morning—Christmas morning—he found his gifts under the *family* tree and a partially eaten cookie left by the true Santa. Apparently, he had been reassured that the fat old jolly guy in the red suit did exist and had his own way of doing things. Our confirmation came when he tracked down his mother after breakfast.

"Mom, does Santa have germs?"

"Why do you ask?"

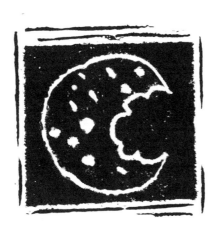

Memoirs of a Geezer Dad

"He didn't finish his cookie and I want to eat the rest of it."
Yeah! Right on, Dude! (No telling what filth he might
have handled in his busy rounds, and no time to wash the fireplace soot off his hands.)

"Go ahead and finish it," my wife said. "I'm sure it's all
right."

He serviced his sweet tooth, and I figured we had a last
believer for one more round of seasons. Then my last child
would outgrow his childhood illusions, and life would
become...well, harder—for us all. The lesson? We should
always yield up our rituals and our faiths slowly and reluctantly,
piecemeal. The heart must soften what the mind will see.

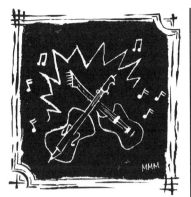

Chapter 12

Culture
Skirmishes

I THOUGHT OF ENTITLING this chapter "Culture Wars," but then realized my two families and I have reduced full-blown wars to mere skirmishes that do not send us off on divergent life paths without ever speaking to one another again. Considering the span of 60 years that separates us all, we are in truly remarkable agreement on what is worthwhile in life and pretty much share the same ethical, political and esthetic values.

Immodestly, I take some credit for that. Living as long as I have has forced me to "grow up"; being a father for over 37 years has forced me to become a peacemaker, hone diplomatic skills, use tact when I clash with my kids over some ethical or cultural issue.

It has been my unscientific observation that most of us are shaped by our time, or decade, if you will. Born in the worst year of the Great Depression, I learned early to want little; and living through World War II as an impressionable and involved child, I found my values—the hard-edged difference between good and evil (and by application right and wrong)—that were later tempered by a tolerant pragmatism picked up as an American university student.

My wife is a Baby Boomer, confident, happy, generous, inclined to luxury, a consumer deluxe, which puts a small gap between us. My first family of sons are Gen-Xers, born in the 1960s, but only tenuously linked to what they think of as a

Memoirs of a Geezer Dad

romantic time they missed out on; they are principled, hard-working, but also self-indulgent spenders. The gap spreads to a chasm.

Then there's the latest batch, children of the late-80s, early-90s, born into a polarized Postmodern world of haves and have nots, where opportunities and possibilities for the favored are offset by highly structured lives that force an intricate balancing act among homework, gymnastic lessons, and soccer or baseball or basketball practice on weekday evenings. Contrast all that with my free boyhood days of benign neglect, and you have social tectonics making a wide valley of a mere generation gap.

This was driven home to me when my daughter Molly, a pre-teener then but looking to her own future no doubt, asked, "Dad, when you were a teenager, did you like rock 'n' roll?"

My answer was atypical of today's parent. "Molly, when I was a teenager, there was no rock 'n' roll."

I was prepared to describe to her Swing and the Big-Band Era and the appeals they had for my generation and me. But she didn't seem either surprised or in need of an explanation. Probably like me asking a miraculously resurrected Shakespeare where he got his ground chuck or what the state of plumbing was in his London. Would our lives be better for knowing the answers?

A couple of weeks later, my thoughtful daughter returned, apparently fishing for a reason to delay doing her homework. "Dad, when you were a kid, did you watch a lot of television?"

"No, Molly, when I was a kid there was no television." I expected her to voice amazement. She didn't. I was about to add how at her age I came home from school, did my homework (hurriedly, but I wouldn't tell her that), and *then*, after an afternoon bowl of Shredded Wheat, listened to 15-minute radio installments of "Terry and the Pirates," "Jack Armstrong, the All-American Boy" and "Captain Midnight"—the three

late afternoon radio serials I remember that united the youth
of my day. But again she walked away without asking for
amplification. Was that good? Bad?

I don't know for sure. But I believe that, ironically, even
paradoxically, generational distance lends perspective, which in
turns fosters understanding. Akin to the bond between grandparents and grandchildren. A bond subject to straining, I readily admit. Don't believe for a moment that our family is free of
the frictions and fallings-out that season normal daily life. The
major rift has to do with money and its spending. As a child of
the Depression, whose father leaned on a shovel for the WPA,
I learned early that frugality was a virtue. A penny saved is a
penny earned, waste not, want not—all those fine old saws
were heaped on me and have stuck in my mind as practical wisdom ever since. All those who have come after me are spend-
thrifts, summed up in that most contemptuous epithet, *consumer!*

I don't see myself as a skinflint, but as a Henley kind of
guy—master of my fate, captain of my soul, the complete existential man who shapes his own destiny with minimal obligations to either environment or heredity.

Then I hear myself angrily holler, "Who left the lights on?"
when seven rooms are lit and six of them are unoccupied.
"Have you people looked at the electric bill lately?" I sound
just like my father…who was also shaped by both nature and
nurture.

Okay, I'm stingy. The three sons of my first family referred
to me as "penny-pinching Dad." Guilty as charged. A friend
at the time—this when Iron Eyes Cody had a TV spot shilling
for the environment—upped the ante to a nickel when he
observed that I "squeezed the buffalo so hard" I "made the
Indian cry." He thought it a clever jibe. I accepted it as an
unmeant compliment.

Memoirs of a Geezer Dad

So what's wrong with buying a new car every ten years? Smart, I'd say. And what's wrong with a few mend marks on your sweatshirts...or even smallish holes in your socks if your Baby-Boomer wife has misplaced her darning egg?

On a recent Tuesday my hard-won frugality collided head-on with this profligate, self-indulgent age. "Please take the van to the car wash today," my wife said as she left for work.

"No, I'll wash it," I said.

"No. I want a thorough, professional job. I'm taking a load of Girl Scouts to the mountains this weekend, remember?"

My temper flushed my face. I hadn't forgotten. But the only time you take a car out for the "$19.95 wash-and-clean-with-fill-up special" is when you're going to a wedding, a funeral, or picking up the Pope at LAX. I was about to remind her of this when I instead bit my tongue. I didn't want to initiate one of those domestic rows that take forever to settle.

Wait for her to go. Then defy her. Let the last guy on the block who still mows his own lawn (so okay, it looks it) show her how "thoroughly" a vehicle can be cleaned and polished—without the industrial-sized vacuum cleaners and banks of water-wasting nozzles the "pros" use.

I didn't rush into the work after she drove off. It was only fair to see her side of the story. She would start by saying that my time was worth more than what I'd spent washing it myself. Soft-soap. If the truth be known, and I took my lifetime earnings and divided by the hours worked, I'd probably come out with 37 cents an hour.

Then there was the bigger picture. "Macroeconomics," the bean counters and sorters like to call it. So my only graduate school C was in that dismal subject. I still know vaguely how it works...how the key is money flow...keeping money circulating and consumers consuming and workers working—even if it means we do each other's laundry. Yes, in the information age service industries have supplanted the smokestack. The haves who sit on their capital are the only villains in the piece.

I took the van in to AAA Deluxe Auto Wash for its over-due cleansing, but in defense of principle only tipped the water-bead-blotterer two bucks. (To those tempted to brandish the word "cheap" I would again counter with "frugal.")

Had I caved in to the persuasive economic argument? I don't think so. Had I done it just to avoid a spat with the little woman? A factor, no doubt. Mostly, though, it was a case of taking the easy way out. It's been a long hard hike getting from the Great Depression to the New Millennium while carrying my burden of virtues, and I just need my rest breaks.

Fewer clashes occur on the culture front. But they do occur and have done so for as long as I've been a parent—a parent of long-held, strong views on this most important subject. I should state up front that my origins are blue-collar, and I've spent my life climbing the cultural (not the economic) ladder. Early on the way up I abandoned pop culture for what is called in textbooks "High Culture."

Many of us have a brief period in our lives when chance and the choices we make conjoin to point us to our futures and determine who we will become. My formative window was late 1954 to late 1955 when I turned 22 in the United States Air Force. I had returned from an enlightening two years based in Japan, where I got a glimpse of how big the world was and the enormous size of my own ignorance, and was sent to a base in rural northern Florida, where segregation was in full bloom, and the white natives were still fighting the Civil War. I hated the place. So much so that when an air-man in my outfit with a pregnant wife got orders for Libya, I

Memoirs of a Geezer Dad

volunteered to go in his place. My buddies hooted. I was crazy
to volunteer to go to such a God-forsaken plot of desert land-
scape.

With the bravado that belongs to the young and foolish, I
promised them, "I won't be there long." I was right. But I did-
n't land in Germany or France as I had hoped. Instead, I was
transferred to Lages Field in the Azores. With time on my
hands and little to do on the smallish Portuguese island of
Terciera out in the mid-Atlantic, I enrolled in the local
branch of American International College and there fell
under the influence of the man most responsible for changing my life. His name was David Morton, a poet and a former editor at more than one New York publishing house, who
had a weak heart and was scraping out a living teaching literature to a captive lot of restless, cooped-up troops. He
claimed he saw something literary in me, and soon enough he
was dealing me books after class to read in my ample spare
time. His only condition: that I come back to him and tell
him what I thought. Responses got me more books to read—
such various and wondrous works as Knute Hamsen's *Growth
of the Soil*, Dostoyevsky's *Brothers Karamazov*, and Anatole
France's *Penguin Island*, among other classics. I was hooked,
and he was pleased. In November of 1955 I was transferred
to Greece; his heart gave out shortly after and he died. To
this day he is my greatest culture hero, my most generous
mentor.

A second, similar epiphany overtook me on Terciera. I
was part of a 20-man weather detachment moved into ten
rooms of a refurbished barracks. Because we had one detest-
ed guy—call him Sleepy Jim—in the outfit, it was decided
we'd draw lots to see what poor wretch would have to share
a room with him. As fate would have it, I got the unlucky
draw, and, amidst the jeers of my good buddies, I moved in

with the priggish pariah. Jim, chaste and a teetotaler, never missed a chance to let us know he considered himself superior to the rest of us—morally, intellectually, and culturally. To the room we shared Jim also brought a new record turntable and his collection of classical music records which, puffing serenely on his pipe, he would silently listen to hours on end. Of necessity, so did I.

Living with Jim for seven months didn't improve my mind or my morals any, but I must admit that he changed my musical tastes. Why, this stuff got better each time you heard it! Better even than Nat King Cole and the Big-Band sound of Ray Anthony! Yes, I was infected, permanently, terminally. When transferred back to Libya in the spring of 1956, I went to the airbase theatre and viewed, along with a mob of rowdy airmen, Bill Haley's *Rock Around the Clock* flick. The troops went absolutely wild, refusing to leave the theatre after the first showing was over, witnesses, it has been suggested by at least one small-time historian, to the birth of Rock 'n' Roll. The melee left me puzzled. What was all the commotion about?

I left the Air Force and entered UCLA, already a devotee of High Culture and dedicated to doing missionary work for the arts. Armed with a convert's zeal, an education in the humanities, and a like-minded wife, I launched a cultural blitzkrieg on my three young sons born in the 1960s. An outgrowth of an overexposure to the high arts was my routine trashing to my kids of American popular culture as some giant, sewage-settling pond, offering little worth adding to Western Civilization's treasure chest. I brushed aside my sons' feeble arguments rooted in esthetic relativism; after all, nobody in their right mind would say Beethoven was a lightweight, Picasso couldn't draw, Shakespeare was an overrated dramatist, or Yeats was a lousy poet. And I had amassed a pretty nice little library to prove it. The richness was all around them—in their own home! All they had to do was open their eyes, ears, minds!

How well did the campaign go? Well, perhaps I was a bit heavy-handed...got ahead of myself. Moreover, as children born in the 60s, my three sons seemed to have picked up that virus that incites resistance and rebellion. Take, for example, my oldest son Eric. When he was a newborn I would steal into his room at night and play, barely audible to his tender ears, tapes of Beethoven's symphonies all night long so that he would absorb the stuff of genius by some kind of sleep-teaching osmosis. Did it work?

Well, he grew up to invent the air guitar, become a Deadhead, and after Jerry Garcia passed on to his reward, write songs for his own rock group, Sancho. I applaud his musical talent...though I guess I'd have to admit that the glass is half empty—no, two-thirds empty—and that pop culture managed to flourish right alongside the high-toned variety, right there in my own first family.

Eric's brothers, the twins, got the same cultural bombardment and went more his way than mine, I must admit. Kurt's heavy metal tastes ran to The Scorpions and Black Sabbath, while brother Karl formed his own rock band, and to this day makes guitars as a hobby. I haven't given up, though. Every Christmas without fail I give each of them (and their wives) classical CDs I think they ought to like. Occasionally, I even find shreds of evidence that they listen to them.

Increasingly, I find other signs that my preaching had some long-range effect. Eric subscribes to *Esquire* and *The New Yorker*. Karl has developed a passion for Steinbeck's work. And Kurt recently got a tenure-track position teaching English at a community college, where he touts the achievements of Donne, Hemingway, and Kazantzakis to his students.

Culture Skirmishes

But overall, I've done somewhat better with my second family. Though I retain my self-anointed Commissar of Culture title, my methods over time have shifted from authoritarian pronouncements to subtle manipulations. Ever since the second batch were infants I've had at least three radios in the house going simultaneously, tuned variously to National Public Radio out of Santa Monica (for news and intelligent talk) or National Public Radio out of Pasadena (for even more news and intelligent talk), KUSC (non-commercial classical music), and KMZT (as in Mozart—a commercial classical music station). Kind of a culture-war equivalent of carpet-bombing. Books and quality magazines are scattered everywhere and talked about aloud by my wife and me. Occasionally, I even deliver poetry readings at the dinner table.

Call it cultural Sensaround…and a subtle preventative. I've learned that each generation needs its own sounds and words and icons to define itself, to separate itself from what's perceived as the dull clowns who have come before. So indoctrination must be indirect.

Direct, too. My wife and I decided to take Molly to a chamber music concert at the Orange County Performing Arts Center when she was five, prompting perplexed looks from the ushers and usherettes who were sure she would disturb the exquisite proceedings with whining or feet-scuffing or some other disruptive kid noises. Confirming our hunch, she didn't. She sat quietly attentive through a piano and violin duo's performance of works by Mozart, Beethoven, Ravel, and Haydn. When it was over and I asked her which one she liked best, she said, "The second one."

Ha! Beethoven wins this round.

Just the other day I was reassured that Molly continues in her highfalutin ways when I asked her what her favorite piece

Memoirs of a Geezer Dad

of music was. Something by *NSYNC? Britney Spears? No, Beethoven's *Seventh Symphony*. Bravo! I do believe that in Molly I have a natural born culture vulture and a successor to my position of family Commissar of Culture when I am relieved at last (at long last?) of my duties.

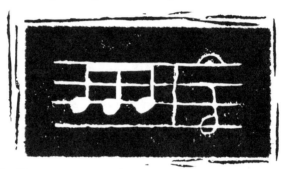

Lately I've seen some hopeful signs with young Franz, too. He doesn't say much one way or the other about the background music he's exposed to daily. But when he does it's similar to last week when he casually asked of a horn concerto warming the kitchen, "Isn't that by Mozart?" Ah! Glory be! Indeed it was.

Madeleine in the middle remains the child beyond my missionary reach. While she tolerates the ambient sound, she will, when the coast is clear, play her CDs with the bubblegum beat. I grumble, but I also give her a generous time window within which to satisfy her plebian tastes.

If I survived Def Leppard and Black Sabbath last generation, I suppose I'll get through the Back Street Boys this time. And yet, there are billions of people—excluding my dearest Madeleine, I'm happy to say—who will go to their graves without having heard Vaughn Williams' *Fantasia on a Theme of Thomas Tallis* at least 50 times. That saddens me.

So much for soothing savage beasts. Everybody knows that books, magazines, CDs, and radio stations are only peripheral scuffle-fields in the struggle between cultures high and low. Everybody knows that center court, center ice, the main event in the culture combat is that boon and bane of the late twentieth century and early twenty-first century—television. Decades after Newton Minnow branded it a "vast cultural wasteland," television is—blame a downright Malthusian increase in channels and signal delivery systems—a much vaster wasteland, relieved by only a few scattered oases.

Of course, one man's oasis is another man's desert. And vice versa. If only I could slake my thirst with the old tried-and-true PBS watering spots—*Nova, Frontline, Masterpiece Theatre*, and those pop concerts watered down in Boston. But age brings with it passivity, and this geezer finds himself more and more in need of "veg" time. Increasingly I collapse into the strategically placed La-Z-Boy to watch old movies, college basketball games, college football games, most Major League baseball games, and any and all dinosaur dig shows, when my faithful viewing companion Franz camps in my lap and lectures me on what we're seeing. (Praise evolution for dinosaurs!)

How do I get all these programs? You guessed it. I have satellite, with its hundreds of gratuitous channels. How do I justify such a cultural lapse? Well, reception in my area is so bad that I must pay to get almost everything in order to get anything. As you might imagine, this poses serious problems for the parent attempting to screen out the graphic depictions of amours that seem obligatory in most contemporary films—serious, exploitative, and just plain bad—and the more corrosive scenes of violence that creep into shows you'd least suspect. Add a second television set stashed in a back room to lessen nasty fights rooted in programming conflicts, and your monitoring time gets stretched. Sure,

Memoirs of a Geezer Dad

one can, and I do, set watching hour limits. But enforcing them is another matter—particularly when you leave the house to shop for groceries or to gas the van.

So constant vigilance yields to spotty censorship. Even then you must pick your fight. Pop culture's hold on the vast wasteland can't be attacked frontally—it's too firm and mighty for that. But you can nibble at its flanks and make snide remarks to nearby ears when marginal material is being watched. That's the tactic I used with the Mighty Morphin Power Rangers, that cynical, mindless, violent slop that only a Philistine like Newt Gingrich could hype. I muttered belittling comments as I passed through the viewing area, questioning the intelligence and moral judgment of its creators. In about six months, the Power Rangers bored their way off the tube, passing out of TV existence locally.

Another spin is to show interest in their choices of commercial fare, providing it's generally harmless and well done. That's why I might pause to briefly watch with them a few minutes of *Rocky and His Friends*, recalling the salutary influence Jay Ward's witty creations had on my first family. This second time around I've even allowed my kids to convert me to background chuckling while they laugh their way through *The Simpsons*; an appreciation of satire always helps make life bearable.

The preferred tactic, however, remains early conditioning to quality, which to me has always meant Public Television, with *Mister Rogers' Neighborhood* and *Sesame Street* for starters. And habitual parental viewing of PBS bolsters this head start for kids. But as children grow older they discover through channel surfing or from their peers an endless menu of junk shows waiting to divert them, pacify them, make consumers of them; combating these is an impossible, full-time job, even for a vigilant, stay-at-home dad. The struggle comes to a focus on control of the remote control, also known in our pad as the clicker, the switcher, or the damn thing!—as in "who took the *damn thing?!*" Possession of that cursed little device gives gatekeeper's powers and brings out the devious worst in everyone.

For example, Mom and Molly departed on a recent Sunday to do their favorite thing—shop. Left alone, without my adult buffer, I knew I was ripe for the con. I was just settling into the La-Z-Boy to watch the NBA on NBC when Madeleine approached from the left flank. "Dad, can I have the front TV?"

"Take the back, honey. Dad's got a Laker game."

"But, Dad! I want to watch *Romeo and Juliet!*"

I'm staggered...my knees are buckling. "You want to watch *Romeo and Juliet?*" I repeat incredulously. Her face lets me know that she knows she's dealing from the strength of my guilt. Could it be the Zeffirelli production? Is she old enough for that? Or is this just a clever bid for control of the control.

"What channel is it on?"

Maddy gives me the number, and I switch to it. Turns out it's a cartoon version, so I can't say no on grounds of it being beyond her ken. And even if it were, could I really deny her request for Shakespeare, even in a chopped, bowdlerized version?

"Doesn't Romeo get dead?" Franz pipes in. He is less inclined toward tragedy, preferring no unhappy endings, thank you.

"Would you like to watch the basketball game instead?" I ask, thinking his choice should be considered.

"No, I want cartoons."

"Saturday was yesterday," I tell him. "This is Sunday."

"Dad," he reminds me. "We have the dish."

Memoirs of a Geezer Dad

Yes, we do. That means the Cartoon Network and *Nick at Nite* and Nick by Day and Nick at Twilight and Nick in the Wee Hours....

Caught in the act, I cave in. Basketball must bow to the Bard. So the Lakers would have to win without me...which they have done before.

I tried to feel virtuous underneath my disappointment. What's more important, after all? Your daughter being introduced to Shakespeare? Or watching a bunch of overpaid jocks run up and down the court in a game you won't remember in a week? Obvious choice.

Not to Franz. "Why don't I ever get the TV?"

"You will in time."

"What time?"

"A fairly distant time. You're an active young boy. You should be getting some exercise anyway."

"What about you?"

A dart in the heart. What indeed. I couldn't tell him that as you grow old you lose energy and become an easy mark for a medium aimed at the tired, the weak, the passive.

"You can watch your cartoons in the back, Franz." (That postage-stamp sized set challenged my waning sight, anyway.)

"Okay," the boy said with excess resignation.

All feelings of nobility for yielding control of the two sets vanished over the next few days. I had done the right thing, hadn't I? But it didn't feel right. I felt wronged and brooded about it for a day. Then, eureka! Professor, get proactive...heal thy own. There and then I decided to seize the sorry medium for noble purposes. Hadn't I shown to my university students videos from the great American Short Stories series with much success in my university literature courses? Secured those videos from my own nearby municipal library? For a dirt-cheap, two-night rental fee of $1.07 per video?

Why not expose my children, ready or not, to the likes of Sherwood Anderson, Henry James, Stephen Crane, Willa Cather, Ernest Hemingway and Flannery O'Connor? Edification on the cheap with some of the greatest short stories ever written! Thus was launched Larry's Masterpiece Theatre. My wife told me I had come into my own as a caregiver.

Tuesday night's premiere showing of Sherwood Anderson's "I Am a Fool," starring a boyish-looking Ron Howard, was preceded by a brief lecture from Dad. I explained to my reluctant audience—there on the threat of a loss of unspecified privileges—that this was a tender, bittersweet, coming-of-age story set in early twentieth century Kentucky. Then I pressed "play," and the reel rolled. Mulish Madeleine looked away during the whole 38-minute showing and said nothing. Franz likewise said nothing but attentively took in the whole thing; probably working on his critical review. Molly complained about it mostly because she was embarrassed by the naiveté of Andy, the story's youthful protagonist who lost the girl of his dreams by posing as someone he was not. "That was the author's intent," I explained. But it made no difference. She didn't like it.

Undeterred, I gave them a day to digest what they had seen and then darkened the living room for a showing of Thursday night's feature. It was Henry James' "The Jolly Corner." Not a very jolly reception, however. Madeleine slipped away within the first two minutes; I think I heard Lisa Simpson's muffled voice from the backroom television. Franz lasted less than a minute longer before sneaking away to his room and the waiting Legos.

Memoirs of a Geezer Dad

Before we were five minutes into James' subtle ghost story, Molly threw a major fit, begged to be excused, and was. My wife and I sat through the last picture show on Larry's Masterpiece Theatre in a funk of failure.

Maybe I had got ahead of myself again. Made a mistake in my choice of author. Henry James was a hard sell to me when I was a college sophomore. So maybe...yet Molly had literary talent and it should be nourished. Trouble is, and she correctly identified it, she likes to read things that make her happy. And literature, I must admit, rarely does. Rather, it stirs the passions, brings tears with its revelations of our imperfect natures and the inscrutable complexity of life. It holds the mirror up to nature and forces us to see what we'd rather not. I understand all that, but still....

Maybe next year, I'll try again. Hand out free popcorn. And certainly not begin with Stephen Crane's "The Blue Hotel." The important thing was I had planted a seed that could flower in the future. Beauty is truth, truth beauty...and the truth will out. Literature says so.

The correlation between culture and politics may not be one-to-one, but a man or woman's cultural stance does play give-and-take with his or her political views...if he or she has any, of course. Maybe it's a survival adaptation born of American get-along pragmatism, but we're not considered a very political people. Oh sure, we have our true believers left and right (but mostly right) and an equal number who catch a quadrennial low-grade fever and put bumper stickers on their cars. But the majority remains distant from the fray, apathetic in the minds of civics scholars who deplore the continuing fall-off in folks who go to the polls.

I'm in a much smaller minority of Americans who take every election seriously. "If the ballot choice is between Heinrich Himmler and Joseph Goebbels for city council," I

am prone to lecture anyone who will listen, "you are obligated to study the men and the issues and make a choice." When
I lived in Los Angeles I was branded by friends a "militant
centrist," a reasonably accurate parsing of my political views,
I must admit. But transplanted to Orange County, where the
whole political spectrum is skewed 90 degrees to the right, I
am unmistakably a liberal—making me an endangered species
who can be hunted without a license in an election year.

Such a social climate puts the dissenter on constant guard.
I have vivid memories of attending one of my daughter
Molly's grammar school open houses and overhearing an over-
civilized gentleman, early middle-aged and slightly paunchy,
tell another parent that he was "a liberal and a pacifist and
therefore—" before his voice was drowned out by ambient
chatter. I wish I hadn't missed this valiant man's grand con-
clusion. And when I left I was tormented by guilt that I had-
n't personally escorted him safely to the Los Angeles County
Line.

Meaning? That I have to be careful of what I say around
my fellow citizens and vent my strong feelings on issues in the
privacy of my home, where I have a habit of directing loud
obscenities at certain politicians appearing on the TV screen,
even when there are young ears near to offend. Can't help it.

The passion may trace to my boyhood and a cold
November day in Cleveland in 1940. My mother had just
months before transferred me from nearby Saint Mary's grammar school in the Slavic ghetto to more distant Saint Joseph's
grammar school in the Irish ghetto; she didn't like the accent
I'd picked up in the first grade.

Walking to my new school took me past Five Points, a
rather prominent local landmark where five major avenues
met at a common focus. Snow had obviously come early that
year, for on that fateful November day, shoveled next to the

Memoirs of a Geezer Dad

sidewalk, were mounds of the no-longer-white stuff—the grainy kind of snow that's been on the ground long enough to absorb soot and get really abrasive. A good supply of same was on hand when I approached the Five Points crossing with a straggle of other young scholars. I noticed ahead three big kids—bullies—forcing the kids into a single file, stopping them, and then questioning them before letting them pass. As I got closer, I heard the challenge.

"Who are you for? Roosevelt or Wilkie?"

"Roosevelt." The boy third in line in front of me was allowed to go on.

"Who are you for? Roosevelt or Wilkie?"

"Roosevelt." A girl in red hood and mittens got permission to move along.

"Who are you for? Roosevelt or Wilkie?"

"Roosevelt." The short guy in front of me got free passage.

"Who are you for? Roosevelt or Wilkie?"

Meek as I was in those days, I still harbored a contrary streak that demanded a voice. I felt sorry for this guy Wilkie, who happened to be from my Mom's hometown.

"Wilkie."

The bullies set upon me and proceeded to wash my face with the dirty, icy snow. Faced rubbed red and raw, I bawled all the way to Saint Joseph's. (Mom sent me back to the Slovenes and Croats the following year.)

I learned my lesson. I haven't voted for a Republican since.

"Since" has meant voting in every election since reaching voting age, save one, when I moved briefly to Colorado from California, couldn't meet residency requirements, and didn't vote at all. That smirch on my citizenship grade bothers me still.

Culture Skirmishes

Out of respect for the democratic process, I don't allow myself to vote often on election day, but I do vote early. That means being up at the crack of dawn with my sample ballot pre-marked and an appearance at the precinct just a few minutes after eight, when the polls open. Why so early? Because I want to do my duty in case I have a stroke or am accidentally killed by a runaway beer truck. True, I live only a half-block from the fire station that serves as my voting precinct, and I have only one street to cross. But I want to make sure that if the worst happens, my last act on earth will have been to vote against every Republican on the ballot. In Orange County, that can be a major undertaking.

I also make a point of taking one of the kids with me when I walk to the voting booth. Why not introduce Molly, Maddy, then Franz to good citizenship early? I notice the precinct workers cock their ears and listen—even chuckle softly—as I field the kids' questions in hushed tones, as though we were in church:

"Yes, Molly, you punch a hole through the card next to the candidate's name, then you turn the page to a new list of candidates."

"Yes, Maddy, anybody in our neighborhood can vote here—but only if they're old enough and registered."

I felt good about my on-the-spot civics lessons. Until the most recent general election, when my companion was Franz the unpredictable. I had just pulled the white cotton privacy sheet around me and inserted my ballot in the plastic jacket when his loud boy's voice pierced the uneven hum of voters and poll watchers shuffling their papers:

"Dad, is Saddam Hussein a Republican?"

Utter silence. You could have heard a voting stylus drop.

Instinctively I knew I'd been presented with the greatest opportunity I'd ever get to display my wit before an audience of more than 20 sets of waiting ears. And I botched it. After too long a hesitation, I stammered, "No, he's an Iraqi…he's got his own party."

I thought I heard a collective sigh of relief…or was it disappointment?

Whatever, the perfect riposte eluded me then, as it does now, bobbing out there in the Platonic ether, taunting me.

It is a question that still pops into mind during idle hours driving the Mojave Desert where I might hope for a revelation from heaven. Maybe it's just a Zen question.

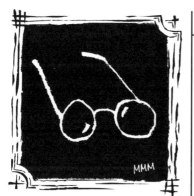

Chapter 13

Kitchen Matters

MAYBE MY FATHER was right about my being a mama's boy. My mother spent almost half her life in the kitchen cooking up good things, and while I don't want to brag, I'm pretty handy there myself. Not to mention being a wise shopper for the groceries that get used there.

My mother was not a gourmet cook. No, her cuisine was quite middle-America, starch-heavy, with an admixture of imports from the German kitchen that a Depression budget and World War II rationing would allow. Her sauerbraten and beef roulade were tasty, if overcooked. Her Ball-jar canned fruits and vegetables and jellies were welcome during the winter months and almost seemed worth those hot summer days spent canning, when steam would rise from bubbling kitchen pots everywhere you looked, and the sweat flowed freely. Her lard-assisted dumplings and potato pancakes were delicious, but she saved her best efforts for baking all manner of cakes and pies and struedels and rich Christmas breads. Still an enduring vision for me is her cinnamon roll dough swelling into white billows atop the winter radiator, proof for a marveling boy of the magic of yeast.

That said, I like to think I've improved on my mother. No, I'm not passing myself off as a gourmet chef, either. No way. (Never could solve the problem of getting all the dishes to ready themselves at the same time, for one thing.) But after 40 years as a chip off the old *hausfrau*, I've become a passably good cook of wholesome, well-rounded, healthy family meals, faithfully absorbing and generally implementing all the dietary wisdom that nutritionists have dispensed in the daily newspaper since my mother's day.

In fact, I call my meals downright tasty…even if that opinion is not always shared by an unappreciative clientele that puts hot dogs at the top of its want list on those rare occasions when we dine out. These same untrained palates haven't yet learned that asparagus is the noblest vegetable of all, with the artichoke a worthy runner-up. My most valued vindications come when a son from my first family dines with us and, appreciative at long last, tells his half-siblings to enjoy Dad's cooking while they can. I like to hear those tributes most when their wives are out of earshot.

Of course, under the grinding daily pressures of keeping a house (admittedly, not very well), I've likewise learned how to cut corners and keep it simple most of the time, as in baked chicken, potatoes and gravy or rice, a fresh vegetable, a salad. On occasions, though, I go the extra spice. My chicken and sausage with navy bean *cassoulet* is much talked about. And my chili usually gets raves, with requests for my recipe. (Which I can't give because I change it every time I make it and can't remember what I have added or subtracted.)

Through trial and error, I've learned to do a pretty good job with fish, as well. Because I know what a preferred source of protein it is, I've worked extra hard to learn how to cook it just the right amount of time and give it the sauce aid it often needs. Some days, though, my drive to serve tasty and nutritious meals clashes with my penchant for saving money. It's almost always when I buy fish from the marked-down table. If I don't prepare it that very evening, delay a day and then cook it the next and serve it to my wife, whose legendary sense of smell places her in the bloodhound league, she will say, "You're going to *eat* that?"

Kitchen Matters

Implied in her inflection is that she will not.

"What's wrong with it?"

"You can't *smell* it?"

I remind her that I haven't lost a diner yet. But often as not, I toss my own serving as well and wallow in guilt over the waste…until I organize my next shopping jaunt when I can recoup my losses.

Armed with detailed shopping lists and coupons in my wallet organizer, I make a tight-circle, three-market route—no more than a mile and a half total driving—to pounce on loss-leader specials and pick up at the lowest possible price such staples as Herdez Medium Salsa, Padrino's Reduced Fat corn chips, and Rosarita Non-Fat refried beans. (I love to heat the beans in the micro for two minutes, add two tablespoons of Newman's Hawaiian pineapple salsa to three tablespoons of the Herdez, mix, and serve as a dip for chips—*que buena!*) If I don't save 30% off the items' regular list prices, I've had a bad day.

Are my good deals financed with coupons alone? No, I am also a raider of the dented can bin, where my tight-fisted tendencies bring coup after shopping coup. When my daughters importune me with fears of botulism, I reassure them: "Not a single case reported in 40 years."

I also do lunches. Not being part of the junk-food generation, and by nature cheap and viscerally resistant to paying exorbitant prices for food I can cook better, I prepare lunches for wife and kids even as I'm cooking their morning breakfasts.

My wife's associates, with whom my better half shares her gourmet *dejeuners*, tell her I should open my own sandwich service for office-bound, pink-collar workers. But they don't understand. I'm not a professional. I do it for love. My secret? Have on hand a variety of flavored breads and then match them with the meat, fish or cheese your instincts tell you are complementary, apply a thin slather of tapinade or garlic butter

Memoirs of a Geezer Dad

or (that old standby) mayo, and viola...you have a stringed instrument worthy of a Heifetz.

Being *meister* of the kitchen poses some truly gnarly challenges. Planning menus is perhaps the most frustrating. Children have a way of insisting on a food one month and refusing to sniff at it the next. Over and over I make the Depression-trained hoarder's mistake of laying in a short ton of some item, only to have it suddenly fall from favor. My hard-won advice? Avoid an oversupply of anything except toilet paper. I still have half a freezer of Hot Pockets awaiting an eater six months after purchase. Then there was the recent dried-fruit binge (and subsequent boycott) that has left me with bags of dried apples and pears and apricots cluttering the pantry. I've toyed with the idea of trying them in a pie or cobbler, but baking is where I fall far short of my mother's mark.

Fresh in family memory and a prompt for snickering is my peach pie fiasco. My son Kurt brought me a pail of the ripe fruit from his tree, and I, against my better judgment and knowing the end result was not worth the kitchen mess, decided to bake a pie from scratch...except for Betty Crocker's assistance with the dough. At first, the batter seemed too dry, then too wet after I added water, then too sticky after an alien strain of flour was added so the goo wouldn't adhere to my hands. The sliced peaches looked fine when I dropped them into their doughy cradle, but I worried about how much cornstarch should go in the thickener and felt uneasy when I popped the pie into the oven.

It looked good when I pulled it out. Pie-loving Molly gave it the first taste test and grimaced in pain. "It's that bad?" I asked, cutting myself a small wedge to check. Yes, mouth-puckering awful. I was thinking of calling my son and telling him to cut down his tree when my eye fell upon my pint-size measuring cup: filled with sugar! I had forgotten to add the sugar! Kurt came by later and delivered a pie he made with a shell and glaze purchased from Ralphs, and sugar. Molly found it tasty. I agreed grudgingly.

No, I'm not much of a *patisseur*. But there are bigger frustrations facing this great wannabe chef of California. That's the want of diners for my dinners. When I was a boy in the Great Depression and during World War II, families ate together, talked together, got to know one another—were glued together, if only because there were no other options. That was before both parents had to work, before television, before teachers loaded kids up with homework, before early evenings were given over to socializing one's children through sports, before clubs and scouting took them away from the home for hours at a time.

As my kids grow older, and my wife works harder, I serve fewer sit-down dinners where we're all at the table. This saps my motivation to be a better chef even as age's infirmities catch up with me. Or so say the signs of the times.

I pride myself on being virtually vanity-free. Only my family and closest friends have the merest suspicion that I have a couple. One is wearing glasses. Clark Kent wears glasses.

In my prime, my vision was so good I could hit a 90-mph fastball out of the catcher's mitt. (Of course it resulted in a weak dribbler to first, but that was the fault of my body, not my eyesight.) The blessing stayed with me right into my mid-forties, when I suddenly found the six-point type in the *Daily Racing Form*'s Past Performances section had become a blur. (Sadly, no, it wasn't a sloppy print job.) Since then, it's been an accelerating descent into frustrating farsightedness, necessitating a new pair of spectacles every two years. I hate them, but if I'm to read—for me a life staple—I must wear them. But not for anything else.

My second point of pride, as advertised, is my culinary skill.

Memoirs of a Geezer Dad

On a recent Wednesday night, my vanities collided head-on. As usual, I wasn't wearing my glasses when I went to the cupboard for the Chicken Shake 'N Bake. When I looked at the pale and spotty coating on the cut-up bird I knew something was amiss. I strained to read the package. By mistake I had used the mix for potatoes, not chicken, and it wasn't practical to try to take it off. Then why not supplement the coating with some good, old-fashioned Italian breadcrumbs? Still sans glasses, I went to the back-up fridge in the garage and pulled out the canister and then doused the chicken a second time. Still didn't look right.

I caved in and put on my glasses and found that I had used a four-year-old can of protein powder long abandoned as a supplement for putting weight between my skinny daughter Maddy's skin and bones. What to do? Glasses firmly on, I tracked down the Progresso breadcrumbs and added them to the previous coverings. Not a pretty sight. But who knew—maybe I had blundered into a blended taste treat that would revolutionize dinner time for America's working families.

Maybe not.

"This looks weird," Franz said as soon as I'd served the meal.

"A new batter," I said reassuringly. "I think you'll like it."

"I like your old recipe better," daughter Molly informed me as she devoured her chicken breast straightaway. But I took her appetite as no vote of confidence. She had just that afternoon returned from three days on a student camp-out in the mountains where the victuals were "so-so," according to her tolerant palate. Besides that, of my six children, she is far and away my most receptive diner.

"What's this?" Madeleine demanded in high disgust. I approached her place and looked down at her chicken. A red rivulet was exposed on the pasty-looking surface of the bird's thigh.

"That's just a small vein of blood," I explained. "You know, a bird is an animal just like us. We have veins carrying blood through our bodies, too."

Almost immediately I knew those words would not help me move the chicken.

"Yuck!" Madeleine exclaimed as she pushed her plate away from her chair.

Her brother, having made a mere dent in a drumstick, nudged his untouched thigh to the rear of his plate. "Can I have more potatoes and gravy, please?"

I briefly weighed holding his spuds ransom until the chicken was eaten. But should I really force the issue and possibly have him go to bed hungry? And he had said "please."

"Yes, you can," I said, knowing my sternest test was yet to come when the little woman got home from work.

"Ummm, chicken," my wife allowed as I retrieved her dinner from the microwave and put it before her.

I held my breath. But not for long. Getting a taste past her nose is like trying to get a fastball past Hank Aaron's bat.

She ate her first bite. "What's the breading?" she asked as she started to painstakingly peel it off the Foster Farms breast.

"An experiment," I said.

"Did you like yours?" she asked skeptically.

I explained that I hadn't actually tasted the chicken myself. I wanted to be sure there was enough to go around. I'd also decided to limit myself to the salad, since I was watching my weight and my cholesterol.

Under further vigorous cross-examination I confessed all...right through my series of vision-induced blunders. "I guess I'm going to have to wear glasses from now on while I cook," I said.

Memoirs of a Geezer Dad

She had ploddingly eaten her denuded piece of chicken—I thought it was a breast, she claimed it was a back—and was now slowly peeling off the veneer on the kids' uneaten pieces with a knife. "You can make chicken salad sandwiches for their lunches," she said.

"Good idea."

We both studied the unsightly pile of shredded meat.

"Or give it to the cat," she amended.

It might work. Probably not, though. I'd tried to palm off some rotten sliced turkey on Marie a couple times in the past, and the usually ravenous beggar sniffed it, put her nose in the air, and walked away. Amazing the instinct for self-preservation.

So maybe this once the solution was to waste and worry not. Clearly, though, my day of decision had arrived. Either I start wearing my glasses while cooking, or I should quit my job as chief cook and bottle, dish and pot washer. My gut tells me to go with the latter option; it also tells me that there's not a chance of that happening.

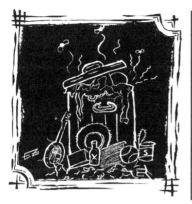

Chapter 14

Living with the Slob Gene

NATURE VERSUS NURTURE. Heredity versus Environment. I've struggled with those classic Western dualisms since I've been old enough to think, my beliefs yo-yoing back and forth between those once-uncompromising poles. Lately though, I've increasingly been drawn toward the Nature/Heredity end of the spectrum, following first the discovery of the DNA double helix, then the unscrambling of the human genome.

All of which leads me to posit the existence of a slob gene and reluctantly admit that I must be double recessive and homozygous for the trait. How do I know this? Pure deduction. My taciturn Lutheran father would always look at *me*—never at my two brothers or my sister—when he solemnly uttered his favorite saw, "Cleanliness is next to godliness." To which I now say (since he is long dead), "Right on, Dad." My three siblings practice what he preached. Enter their homes or their cars and inspect their persons, and they are always squeaky clean and orderly—proving out the 3 – 1 Mendelian ratio favoring the dominant gene. ("You have inherited the cleanliness gene, and I've been left with the godliness one," I like to tell my brothers and sister, who are never amused by my insight.)

I likewise know I'm a slob because all three of my live-in children are slobs. Implicit in that statement is that my wife is at least heterozygous for the trait. But it gets worse. My wife also packs around the packrat gene, shared with some of her sib-

Memoirs of a Geezer Dad

lings who are most generous in giving us the overflow from their collecting. So far my son Franz has tested positive for packrat-mania—enough to kick in the multiplier effect, when clutter accumulates exponentially. The bottom line? When the two bad genes conjoin you get mess-makers who can't throw anything away. You can imagine what a burden all this puts on me as a homemaker.

My wife and I talk about our dilemma regularly. We've formed a kind of ongoing, combination two-person support group/problem-solving task force. Like grownups do. Like good parents should. We've made little progress.

My wife suggested I examine myself and come up with a ruthlessly honest self-evaluation—similar to what I did when giving students a course grade—of my parenting performance and try to improve. I took her advice to heart and came up with this report card:

Role Modeling: .... A^-
(A little less anger and I could raise it to an A.)

Cooking and Shopping: .... B^+
(Could improve with more encouragement and without the thieving dog.)

Caregiving: .... B
(Could do better if I were nimbler and didn't have to write in my journal.)

Sounding Reveille to Four Slugabeds: .... A^+
(A truly heroic and unappreciated effort here.)

Housekeeping: .... D
(A gentleman D at that; closer to an F+, really.)

Yes, my major fault. Unwillingly and unwittingly, I just can't keep a clean house…or a house clean and mess-free. As non-material as I am by nature, I do have a weakness for collecting books. Indeed, they have become my security blanket, lining half the walls in the house. Unfortunately, they are not all on their shelves. I once could say I had read them all; now I'm stretching it to say I've read two-thirds in their entirety, though my intentions remain good. Instead books with marks and magazines crimped to chosen pages where reading was interrupted litter the house, awaiting my return. My wife and kids have picked up the bad habit from me, the end result looking much like a Dresden library circa 1945.

Sensitive to our "collective" shortcomings, I've tried recently to set an example by immediately re-shelving books and boxing magazines—just putting things back and throwing out on first contact junk mail (including the myriad unsolicited catalogs that miraculously find my wife's address).

As part of the same clean-up, I've initiated a clothes standdown, whereby for every garment I buy, two must be relinquished...to Goodwill or the ragbag, depending on condition. I suggested my wife do the same. She's still considering it, I believe. I've even gone so far as to hint, very gently to be sure, that we rent a Public Storage bin to house some of her clothes (including the cheerleader's skirt from junior high) and shoes and hats collected over the last three decades and presently clogging three and a half closets. Touchy subject. No positive results to date.

We both agree that my wife is neat and clean. But she admits to having a hard time discarding things she has collected that please her. Unfortunately, many things please her, and they tend to pile up. Or she puts them in a bag and hangs same from whatever hooks, doorknobs or chair backs might remain unused for the purpose. This practice has earned her locally the tag of "resident bag lady" and added to a household of clutter and disarray.

Further proof that my wife recognizes her problem is her

propensity to collect baskets and trays, which along with bags serve the purpose of holding collectibles. Trouble is, what do you do with the bags, baskets and trays when they all are filled and themselves fill the house to the garage rafters?

Always on the trail of a solution, I've suggested she open a boutique and call it Bag, Basket and Beyond; she has stock enough to trade for years. I meant it as a jest or a bona fide business opportunity idea–she could take it either way. I got a frown for my pains. Apparently her sense of humor matches her entrepreneurial spirit.

To no better result, I've caught the same container/vessel fever. Only I invest in clothes hampers, wastebaskets, and— when they're on sale at the stationer's store—cardboard storage boxes. The sad result? At last count we have six hampers to supplement six clothes baskets in the house, yet a random check shows that at any given time there are as many clothes on the floor or tossed onto sofas, chairs, or hung on doorknobs as occupy hampers, which at best operate at only half-capacity. Wastebaskets? Ten at last count, though only half are in indoor service; the other half have migrated outside to hold dog droppings, kitty litter, mulch-destined trimmings from rose and bougainvillea bushes, and rusty water stains from last winter's rain. As for those more-than-a-score of storage boxes, although some wear such hopeful labels as "Medical Bills" or "Children's School Drawings," most remain empty. I simply don't have the time to go through the piles of paperwork steadily growing vertically from any and all horizontal planes within the house.

The floor, of course, is one such plane. Yes, I confess, crops of paperwork spring from there, too, to become additional hazards for a six-feet, four-inch-tall decrepit arthritic whose neck bones don't hinge well enough to see dangers lurking below knee level. I must already contend with a slatternly family's habit of leaving partially open every dresser, bureau, or side-

Living with the Slob Gene

board drawer—typically at shin level—to show to company a tuft of napkin or a corner of an old postcard or a loop of electrical cord. Amazingly, I'm the only one to notice these untidy flags, and, regrettably, the only one blind and feeble enough to purple his legs on the jutting wood.

As you might imagine, I do not embrace "friends" who just "drop by" unannounced to visit my untidy domain; indeed, on occasion I've actually hidden out and ignored the doorbell, despite the fact that my car is in the driveway. Maybe they'll think I'm on one of those three-mile walks I never take. And I'm particularly sensitive about neighbor ladies and my kids' friends' mothers who drop by to deliver an abandoned baseball glove or a lost Girl Scout sash. To receive such visitors, I require at least an hour's warning to spruce up the kitchen and living room and herd the livestock into the back yard. Without an alert, I just rudely plant my 230-pound bulk in the doorway, while effusively expressing my thanks and trying to kick dirty clothes and dust-balls out of sight.

My wife and I do try to cope with the mess, despite time constraints. She works out of the home in excess of 50 hours a week and needs to rest up on the weekend. Of course, I'm tied up with my daily duties as cook, shopper, transportation provider, journal keeper, and *T'ai chi chih* exerciser—not much time left for either of us to dust the bookcases.

Early on, my wife sold me on hiring a once-a-week housekeeper; it became a hard sell when I imagined myself as a boy trying to convince my father he should hire a Bermuda-grass-pulling gardener. But I caved, and we briefly tried it. We found ourselves working 18 hours straight just to get the house presentable for the house-cleaner service, whose young maids mopped the floor, bleached the sinks, and put foil under our stove burners. Not much else. And not worth the money.

More recently, on those increasingly rare occasions when we

have houseguests, we work so hard just getting the place cosmetically clean that we're too exhausted to entertain properly when they arrive. When guests depart, things go right back to normal, and I find, often as not, I'm the first one to lapse into slovenliness.

My wife still holds on to hope. She keeps bringing up our long-planned add-on that would give us another 500 square feet of living (her word) or storage (my word) space. I, however, who consult the monthly Fidelity brokerage account statements featuring a mostly tech stock portfolio, find myself praying in private for a house fire.

Some might claim my wife and I have only ourselves to blame. "Drop the fiddle and bow and cut with the sob story. You got a mess, you got troops to clean it up. Put your kids to work! Be a proper parent!" Yeah, sure. Easy for them to say. Actually, I'd have a better chance swimming the Hellespont doing the butterfly.

You see, my children think they're above menial labor. No, of course it can't be a right of birth, because I, their progenitor, am a commoner condemned to toil daily in their place. It's just that they truly believe they were meant for better things, such as reading, primping, shooting hoops.

Take Molly, my oldest, whom I have dubbed Dame Lydia Languish. An intellectual virtually from birth and now resolutely embarked on the path to academia, she flat-out considers housecleaning chores beneath her. She has the straight-A report card to push in my face, as if to say, "Would you rather have an honor student or a household slave?" Framed that way, and now that she's in high school acing AP and honors courses that put her GPA well above 4.0, it's a mighty tough choice. Maybe her personal edification *should* come first.

On Molly's behalf, I should say she holds nothing back in her praise of a family member who *does* work. "That's a great job you're doing cleaning the toilet," she will say to me as I'm grinding my glass knees on the bathroom tile floor, short-handled brush in hand. "Even better than the last time." A part of me always feels honored to have such a grand lady take notice of my humble labor; another resents the airs of this bogus duchess who deigns not to dirty her own hands with such nasty business.

Then there's master Franz, the littlest slob (in stature, hardly output) who, as I've mentioned before, has written his own anthem in condemnation of work. Molly first cleverly contracted his initials FLM to "Phlegm," her way of describing his phlegmatic ways when answering the call to labor. It was such a good brand that I soon knighted him Sir Frank Phlegm, like his oldest sister a member of the idle non-working class. He truly is one of kind. He wanders the house and yard in a transcendent cloud, unconsciously shedding in his wake a continuous trail of toys, cast-off garments, partially nibbled snacks, tiny bits of torn paper, toy rocket ships crafted of rusty springs and scraps of foil…the mess defies summation.

I tried long and hard to discipline the little guy. Forget about it. When I send him to his clean room (a jungle I won't enter without a native guide), nothing happens. Even when I threaten to ground him and actually follow through, turning his friends away at the door. Even when I threaten to cancel future ice-cream treats or movie dates…and do. Nothing ever happens. To find out why, I've steered Sir Frank into his trash-strewn room with orders to clean, then periodically returned to peek in at him. The pattern is always the same. He will pick up a first item (maybe a legless toy soldier), add a Pokemon card, then a tarnished plastic battlestar, and he will stare at them, massage them and—poof!—he is transported into some far-off place out of time at play with his imagination, dreaming who knows what.

Memoirs of a Geezer Dad

The pathology became even more tangled recently when he guilelessly confided to his mother, "I feel uncomfortable when my room is clean." How could I possibly punish him? His need to escape the dreary here-and-now calls to mind another stargazing boy who lived a similar life 60 years ago—now grown to a man who perhaps saddled his son with another downside genetic legacy. Besides, who am I to disrupt what might be his breakthrough ruminations on Super String Theory?

My Madeleine, too, has slob credentials, but unlike her brother and sister, and like me, she is bothered by mess. Periodically she gives in to a compulsive need to clean and straighten. When the Red Tornado, as I call her, goes into frenzied action, you had best step aside and keep out of the way of her aggressive wet mop. Basically, though, she's a clearer/stuffer type of cleaner-upper, with the end look one of surface neatness. You can't fault her determination. But you learn to regret these storms that in their wake carry off such things as gas bills, rebate checks, and presumed letters from the Nobel Committee. Where do they go? Probably to share company with those single stray socks, down some tiny local black hole, never to be seen again.

What's a geezer father to do? Learn to live in a pigsty, I guess. Still, it's their lack of embarrassment that bugs me most. How can they walk through or step over filth and never even seem to notice it, then shamelessly invite their friends to step over it with them? I have been known to point to an offending heap and await their shared feelings of disgust. I'm still waiting.

For three years I tried on them the "Shame Game" in which I attempted to appeal to their senses of personal pride. My "real people" spiel included such barbs as, "real people don't eat spaghetti with their hands," and "real people pick their towels off the floor when they're done bathing," and "real people clean their bedrooms at least once a month." It was clear being tagged as fake people did get under their skin. But I abandoned the campaign a year ago when Madeleine lured me into a verbal trap.

"You know my friend Shannon, Dad?"

"Sure. I know Shannon."

"Do you think she's real?"

"Shannon? *Real?* Of course, she's real."

"Well, her room is messier than mine!" Said triumphantly, turning the blade back on its wielder.

Time for a change in tactics. Not long ago I found a cockroach at the bottom of the Maytag washer I was unloading. With such a loathsome teaching aid, here was a chance to drive my point home. I called the kids together in the kitchen. "You know what I found in the washing machine today?"

The veteran pig-farmers waited silently to hear out my latest rant.

"A roach!"

They shuffled, unfazed by the shocker, relieved I think that they were not implicated directly. Then Franz bolted out the front door in a high state of excitement. I heard his pre-pubescent trill pierce the evening air as he called to his neighbor buddy, "Guess what, Brad? We've got a *cockroach* in our washer!" Maybe the neighbors were watching TV with the volume turned up.

Well, at least we keep our roaches clean.

If I had any hope of cultivating a sense of shame in Franz, that was soon dashed. When I went to pick him up from an overnight stay at a friend's house—a visit to be immediately reciprocated at our place—he again let his excitement rule his tongue. He had barely scrambled into the van before bursting out with: "Dad! Guess what? Good News! Danny's house is a mess just like ours."

I couldn't suppress a thin smile through the blush. Call it a

Memoirs of a Geezer Dad

shaky entry into the social world for my youngest son, and make what you will of that. I just hope Danny's mother didn't hear the good news from her doorway.

In the end, I know I have only myself to blame. Whether I gave them a lousy gene or they chose their slobbish ways of their own volition, the buck comes back to me. I am keeper of the trough, after all. Maybe if I spent less time on this journal and more time doing the drudge work of keeping house, the dump might look better, and they might take more pride in keeping it that way. Then again, maybe not. And why waste time scrubbing sinks and toilets when I can be with them enjoying the good times? By way of further mitigation, I can also take credit for passing on to them my godliness gene.

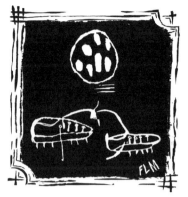

Chapter 15

A Few Things New Under the Sun

To every thing there is a season, and a time to every pur‑
pose under the heaven. And as this geezer's generation
passeth away, and another generation cometh, he findeth there
is a time to laugh and a time to weep. Generally, I laugh on the
good days, which seem shorter this season, and weep figurative‑
ly on the bad days, which seem longer than they used to be.

What's a bad day? Typically, it goes like this: I creak out
of bed with a sudden gout attack that sends me reeling down
the hall like a two‑legged crab and feeling that familiar pain
I've never been able to adequately describe to any non‑suffer‑
er of the disease. It adds to the morning stress of making
breakfast and lunches for our breadwinner and the three bud‑
ding scholars, the younger two of whom find reason to com‑
plain about the food and drop late‑falling homework onto the
kitchen table for correction and/or signature. The young ones
also snipe at one another and dawdle until they are late for
school.

In hurrying to drive them there, I strike my gouty knee
against the car door as I get in—a blow that normally would
elicit a cry of pain and a string of Anglo Saxonisms young ears
shouldn't hear. Instead, I "ooooh" my feeling of relief, because
the pain from the blow distracted me from the pain of the
gout. There at last is my best description!

No sooner do I return from dropping off the kids than I
find a lunch bag left on the kitchen table, necessitating a

return trip to school. Back home again, I see water pooled on the kitchen floor, a sure sign the freezer has failed again and that I will have to spend the next four hours cooking thawing frozen meats that will otherwise spoil. How many chicken breasts can we eat over the next week? How will I vary their preparation?

When I pick up the kids from school, I learn from Franz that he needs a set of crayons immediately or he's going to get an F on an art project. How can that be? I throw away crayon stubs of all lengths and hues every day, and we've still got them scattered all over the house, yard, garage, car—you name it! "Yeah, but they aren't the right color."

Why argue? I detour on the way home to buy the crayons. The cashier, a garrulous woman of about 40, views my cantankerous trio in kinetic action.

"Grandpa's day to have them," she says with a patronizing smile-smirk.

"But they're mine," I say awkwardly, really wanting to disown them on the spot. "I'm their *father*."

She laughs. It sounds halfway between derisive and nasty. Does she doubt me? Pity me? No time or mind to ask. I hurry them home for homework and the start of what for epochs has been referred to as The Children's Hour, that time of late afternoon horror when everyone's nerves are frayed, and tempers are powder kegs with burning fuses...that time when death does not seem so terrible a prospect for an old, weary, and failed peacemaker.

Some call it sibling rivalry. I know the end result as sibling warfare, the inevitable capstone to those typical bad days. With my first family I ascribed it to just having three innately aggressive boys born within 15 months of one another. Now, with a majority of girls in the second wave, I'm aware that gender makes no appreciable difference…except that the progress from crooked look to sharp words to fist on flesh is more drawn out with the gentler sex. I'm tempted to call quarreling a constant of family life, though I can't allow myself the generalization. There are single-child families where the hostility must be internalized or directed elsewhere, I guess.

Other constants are better known. If there are three battlers, two will ally against the third, though alliances can shift at a moment's notice. Usually, shared blood will draw siblings together against a threatening outsider, but if one of your children (most often the oldest) does go over to the "enemy," then be alert to a greater danger of actual physical harm being done. This mere "breach of blood" points to a potentially serious problem.

How does one handle the small-time brawls? I've tried different tactics with limited success. I've played the interventionist Solomon, hearing arguments, acting as a jury of one, only to have my judgments largely ignored. I've tried backing off into relative isolation, letting the combatants work out an armistice on their own, worrying inside that they might do lasting damage to one another, but outwardly saying only that I would call the paramedics if needed, and in case of a fatality, I would appear for the prosecution.

Not much of a deterrent. The only unqualified success I had—and it was temporary—ended a classic clash between Molly and Madeleine. Amid shrieks of pain and the thud of blows I bellowed, "Stop it! You're putting stress on my bypassed heart, and stress shortens my life!"

I had gone too far. Done what I promised myself I would never do…what my dear sainted mother had done to me and my warrior brothers, when, more than once, she said to us in exasperation, "I hope some day you'll remember sending your poor mother to an early grave." She died at 65, of leukemia, and I'm still appealing my self-imposed sentence of third-degree woman-slaughter to myself. Maybe, for her and for me, it comes down to peace at any price.

That's still no excuse for dropping guilt bombs. There are other ways to control, if not eradicate, sibling strife, as many a stay-at-home mom and lately this geezer have learned. It starts with realizing that July is the cruelest month. That's when the dear begotten leave the confines of June's classroom for the summer vacation freedom to really get down to some bare-knuckle combat, expressed in a non-stop medley of nasty words, semi-violent deeds, and just plain orneriness all around. I've learned over two generations of parenting that it's best to keep your heirs busy and separated. That means putting them in as many activities outside the home as possible, while trying to keep them as far apart as possible when they must be inside. (For the latter, after I break up a fight I assign each child a private "cooling off place," where they are to temper their tempers alone, undisturbed. Results? Modestly favorable, though in the heat of summer's battles, apparently, there are no neutral corners.)

My wife first pointed the way toward keeping a part-time peace in a constructive way. In the name of socialization, she enrolled the girls early and separately in pre-school classes and ballet and gymnastics. I built on the idea four summers back when I discovered the concept of the sports camp...or its equivalent. Expensive, to be sure. But a small price to save my sanity. I splurged on a variety of separate-but-equal summer diversions, calculated to put the kids' time to good use and, of course, to keep them out of each other's (and my) way.

For Molly, my oldest, there would be softball (which she had played well enough before), volleyball (an introduction), and a course in creative writing (a field in which she shows promise). Madeleine, already a skilled gymnast, would spend a week at gymnastics sport camp, take a month of swimming lessons to perfect her freestyle stroke, and enjoy an introductory season of softball in the Pixie League.

As for the little guy, there would be a third summer of swimming lessons for dedicated stones (with hopes they would finally get him to the dog-paddling stage), and, prize of prizes, the grail itself, a week-long baseball camp conducted by the local community college coaches. Franz was ecstatic at the prospect.

My crowning achievement was a large and detailed three-month calendar of events posted on the refrigerator door, so all would know who would be doing what at any given time. Of course, I consulted it most, busy as a Tijuana taxi hurrying from drop-offs to pick-ups and sandwiching grocery shopping in between. Not much time left for journal writing. In fact, the whole program was a flat-out hassle. Nevertheless, it beat playing Clyde Beatty, cracking the whip to keep the fang-bared creatures apart in one's own den.

Franz's baseball camp came first in the summer. I confess my eyes moistened when I deposited in the coaches' care the little blond fellow dressed in uniform remnants of the Dodgers and Rockies (his first two Tee-Ball teams), spikes on and batting gloves tucked into his back pocket (like the Major Leaguers do).

Besides being sentimental, I also confess I'm a little bit jealous. When I was a kid there was no Little League baseball. No Babe Ruth League. Only unruly pickup games without coaches and rife with bad habits picked up watching big-bellied, beer-league adults play softball. Softball! Yeah, we played it, too, at the city park, but it was a wimpish imitation of the real thing. We didn't get to play genuine, organized, nine-inch hardball until we got into the American Legion league when we were 15 or 16. American Legion Baseball… the one certifiably positive contribution to American culture made by the organization.

My "Discovery Summer" program worked so well my wife pushed to extend it into the school year and soccer season. Her arguments were persuasive. Part of their continuing socialization, she explained; no reason for them to be as socially deprived as their father had been. With my usual skinflint's misgivings, I signed up our two youngest in soccer for the first time.

I wasn't prepared for the sticker shock. At the elaborate try-out, sign-up ceremony, I paid $75 for nine-year-old Madeleine and another $75 for six-year-old Franz. All that for an eight-week season. Wow! Then again, the fee covered uniforms (wearable for only eight weeks, I guess, unless you wanted to make a radical fashion statement), plus a photo of the team and the player. (More elaborate and costly photo packages were available for an additional payment that I was not prepared to make.)

That was just the first bite. The uniform issued to my petite Madeleine was clearly meant for a full-figured teenager.

"It'll have to be tailored," my wife said.

Tailored! Well, I guess so…I had to have my daughter looking presentable for her debut in Orange County society. The cost? Twenty dollars. Ouch! But then Number 2 did look cute in her Kelly green outfit with a matching bow ($4; none for the lad, thank you) in her red hair.

As for my son, on whom the black and white togs of Team Lightning hung as though he were a junior coat rack, well, I could always hope for another growth spurt.

A Few Things New Under the Sun

Soccer shoes came next. Thirty dollars, times two. Add shin guards—another $8, times two.

Further charges lurked in the greensward. For the team banners—felt scrolls with team symbols and players' names emblazoned (in this case the Peperoncinis and Lightning, respectively)—add another $8, times two.

Plus $20 times two for a pair of AYSO Region 117 discount cards that allowed me to get two fast-food orders for the price of one at participating eateries...not quite what a guy with my cholesterol count puts on his Christmas want list.

Add another $13.50 as our share of sponsorship for a team that couldn't find one.

Still to come were the intermittent *apres*-game pizza parties, BYOV (Bring Your Own Visa), times two.

The tab for two soared to more than $400!

There were no such programs for this Depression-Era kid! Good thing, too, because there was no such money. That $400 would have gone for bread, baloney and coal for the winter...and perhaps a bottle or two of schnapps to see Mom and Dad through the Cleveland cold.

That miserly complaint aside, I must confess to two other reservations about my kids playing soccer. I would be attending their matches, of course. That would mean feigning interest in a sport that for raw viewing appeal I've always equated with watching snails mate. Could I pull it off? Granted, my resistance to the game softened somewhat when the American women won the World Cup. But as a good American who loves baseball, likes basketball, and watches football with diminishing interest as my testosterone continues its long slide downhill, making a place for a boring, simple-minded sport imported from abroad is like breaking up—very hard to do. Perhaps mine is a generational view; certainly, contrary evidence abounds on our playing fields and public parks every Saturday.

Memoirs of a Geezer Dad

My last reservation was literally more down-to-earth: How to watch the games. The Rice Krispies that have long owned my knees are now colonizing my left hip, making it both difficult and painful to plump my 230 inert pounds down on a sideline blanket, as I did the first two matches. My efforts at getting up provided more of a spectacle than anything that transpired on the field of play. For the next two games I tried a low-slung lawn chair. Good as long as I didn't move. Rising, again I looked like the Arthritis Foundation's poster geezer.

Finally I invested in a high-seat collapsible canvas folding chair with arms. Much better. Add another $15 for the chair. Times two with the one for the old lady.

The actual season began inauspiciously enough, with a total of five losses and one tie for the Peperoncinis and Lightning ensemble. It had to get better, I told myself. And it did. Not much, but on one particular Saturday both teams actually won by identical 4–1 scores. I cheered lustily when the Peperoncinis went deep into the playoffs and when my son scored the only goal in his last game. But usually I forgot the scores within a week.

My kids' coaches and the other spectating parents didn't seem to remember them any better. They practiced what the soccer league preached. It mattered not whether you won or lost or tied, but how you played the game…and the fun you had. Nothing like the raucous conduct of parents when I coached Little League Baseball with my first family. And certainly light years removed from the explosive and potentially violent atmosphere that attended the football games two of my sons played back then. Yes, youth soccer as played by seven-through-nine-year-olds in these civilized parts reflects well on coaches, parents, and kids.

But was the season a success? Yes, I guess. New friends were made. Healthy exercise was got. On the other hand, costly precedents were set.

A Few Things New Under the Sun

Worth it, my wife insisted. We should view the success of Discovery Summer, validated by a rump session of autumn soccer, as a paradigm for the future. As she explained it to me, not only would it keep them flush with activities, and lessen sibling conflict, the plan would advantage our children, engage them for a lifetime—might even lead to careers, or at the very least, sustain lifelong avocations. How could I resist? Maybe I could score a second mortgage. Or perhaps refinance.

We have followed the blueprint since, but have learned to stay flexible and live with disappointment when our children change their minds and interests. Molly aggrieved her mother when she gave up ballet, and I moaned over the waste of talent when she announced, after finishing second in the city's 100 meter finals without benefit of a coach or training, her permanent retirement from track and field. But I backed off. I still harbor memories of my father bullying me into playing high school football as a six-feet and one-inch-tall, 158-pound, third-string left-end cleat-mat for single-wing formations running right.

In another non-applauded change of direction, pre-teen Madeleine quit soccer and softball in favor of a class in Hip-Hop dancing. Not a good change, her parents think. On the other hand, Franz quit Pokemon on the Game Boy to became a super sleuth for Carmen San Diego, showing a positively un-American interest in world geography. As I have learned again and again, children, too, have their seasons, and should have a time to choose what vanities they will chase. That's what it's all about, isn't it? Make what you will of the time you're given?

Yet, watching them at their play, I find myself sharing the poet's yearning to freeze time or turn it back. Arrest their growth and reverse my aging.

Not to be. So just squeeze the present for all it's worth.

I repeat that mantra to myself often, but wistfully. It has taken a few years to sort out my feelings. Yes, the times they

have a-changed, and there are some things new (and not necessarily better) under the sun. Childhood—the one they
know—is not what it used to be. Kids are too many now, in too
cramped a space, too rushed, too competitive, under too much
pressure to join or fit in or fall behind or below their "peer
group."

My kids will never know the joys of a freelance childhood
like I had and appreciated too late. Never bask in
neglect…never have the slack time to dream on your own and
drift to wayward until you caught up with yourself and your
contemporaries wading through the same sluggish tide…
never spend your lamb-white days running your heedless ways
down the rivers of the windfall light under the sun that is
young once only.

Okay, adjustments to the budget were made for the catego-
ry I've labeled "Child's Play." Curiously, the monthly tab
roughly matches the total of my monthly Social Security benefit. In order to see that my children meet the new demands of
growing up advantaged, I've pretty much given up Laker,
Dodger, Angel, and Bruin games, as well as deafened myself to
the inveigling whinnies emanating from Santa Anita and
Hollywood Park. That keeps me closer to home where I've
become a faithful spectator at the children's performances and
contests. The admission price is right, and I've already paid for
the bucket chair that affords me close-up viewing.

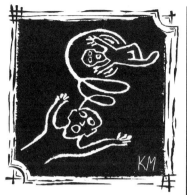

Chapter 16

Fear and Trembling

To me, the greatest grief any parent can know is the death of a child. It's a grief I've been spared, though I've gone through my share of harrowing close calls. And I have friends and acquaintances who lost one (or more, in one case) through accident or disease—a loss that leaves life-lasting scars and has resulted in the ruin of more than one friend's marriage. I continue to live with the fear, and I tremble at the mere thought of it happening to me.

My first scare came early in my first marriage with the birth of twin sons. Kurt weighed in first at 5 pounds 3 ounces, to be followed three minutes later by Karl, who weighed 5 pounds 13 ounces. Jubilation gave way to concern after five weeks when Kurt's weight shot past his twin's, whose actually began to drop at the same time he started regurgitating breast milk in a forceful stream, as though expelled through a nozzle. The phenomenon fit perfectly Dr. Spock's description of projectile vomiting.

In a panic, my wife and I rushed Karl to our pediatrician. The diagnosis was immediate: pyloric stenosis. Pyloric *what?* A congenital obstruction in the duct leading from the stomach to the intestine. Moreover, the doctor prescribed immediate abdominal surgery to save the infant from fatal dehydration. As for that heretofore unknown-to-me condition, it was an abnormal thickening of the muscle between the stomach and small intestine that constricted the passage of ingested fluids and

183

rejected them with such force that a stream of milk went shooting across the room. Our doctor explained it as a gene-carried trait three times more likely in males that, before twentieth century advances in surgical techniques, had long resulted in the early death of largely first-born sons, as old graveyards will attest, if you bother to check the headstones. Today, he assured us, the condition was quite treatable, almost routine.

My trembling hands and churning stomach clearly communicated my skepticism as they wheeled the tiny, bottom-up sleeping infant centered on the huge gurney into the operating room. No margin for error that I could see. So little blood to lose, so little time in which to cut—and cut accurately—and then sew up. I remembered thinking as my son disappeared behind the swinging doors how I had never believed parents who said they would gladly die in their child's place when life hung in the balance. Contrary to human nature, I told myself. Wrong! Now here I was copping that same hackneyed plea that whatever gods there were take me, not my baby.

They took neither. The doctor made the cut, and my son recovered quickly and grew robustly, the only remaining sign of the trauma being the proportionate growth of the original two-inch incision scar over his present six-feet, four-inch, 250-pound frame.

Three years later I had my first scare in the 911 department when his twin Kurt, while exuberantly bouncing in his crib, rammed a sharp bamboo stick through the roof of his mouth. Off to the ER and more fear and trembling. Fortunately, the wound quickly closed and healed, without any lasting speech impairment to the toddler, as we had been led initially to fear.

The last of my sons from my first marriage, Eric, gave me my most terrifying moment when he was 12. I stepped into the backyard patio to see the boy firing up the barbecue by sprinkling a gallon can of gasoline on a bed of smoldering charcoal.

No! My scream lodged in my throat, but my face must have paled to the hue of death, because Eric froze when he saw me, even as the dripping gas trickled from the smoking briquettes to pool on the ground.

To this day, I do not know why the gasoline did not ignite

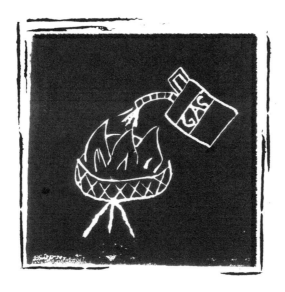

and blow him and me to smithereens. Probably not quite the right mix of petrol fumes and oxygen. In any case, it took me several hours to get my breath and wits working in harmony so I could give my son a tremulous lecture on the lethal properties of gasoline.

Such crises are much easier to handle after the fact, sans suspense, I was to learn one day between university classes. When I picked up my ringing office phone my wife Timarie, with controlled tension in her voice, said, "The first thing I want you to know is Kurt's all right. There's been a backyard accident, and a neighbor boy is in very serious condition. An ambulance has been called." Turned out the neighbor boy was dead when it arrived. My eighteen-year-old son was indeed alive, if shaken. The pair had climbed a tall pine tree in the backyard next door, and the other boy had reached out and touched a high-tension wire that knocked them both out of the tree. A time of much grief, certainly, with attendant legal hassles that dragged on for years. But I'm forever thankful that my wife took the ultimate suspense out of the tragedy, saving me the anguish of sweating out—even for 20 seconds—an uncertain outcome for my son.

All parents know the worry never ends, the fear never ebbs. It actually peaks when your kids reach driving age, and your sleep turns fitful, the churning unconscious mind half-waiting for the dread CHP phone call after midnight. The question begged is, why would anyone go through it all a second time? Grant fear a second front with one generation new to driving and another new to walking? I'm not sure. Maybe the need of family and the company of small children is my great weakness. My way of fending off depression by filling my days with action benefiting others who happen to be my own. How else explain facing another round of paramedic calls and hospital runs, administering those post-midnight baths to get the kid's fever down below 104 degrees, the all-night dozing vigils to log in the time you've spooned out with quaking hands doses of Motrin and Tylenol and antibiotics?

At first I thought it would be easier the second time around because Molly, my first daughter and first child of my second family, was remarkably sound—and has remained so from infancy on, with tubes implanted in her ears to stop infections the only mar to an otherwise clean bill of health. But human failure is always ready to mess up what nature chooses to pass on. I am one of those human bunglers. Even now it is a memory I can only call up with great difficulty, as I'm experiencing at this moment, writing about it 16 years after the near-tragic fact.

Fear and Trembling

It was a warm May afternoon, and I opened the front door to cool off in a cross-breeze while I graded final examinations on the living room sofa. Suddenly I felt a spasm of dread pass through my body. I jumped up and ran down the hallway to check on year-old Molly who was just learning to walk. Not in her room! Not in my room! With a bellow I bolted out the open front door. Just in time to see the toddler, red curls bouncing radiantly in the sun and diaper sagging low, about to step off the curb into a boulevard busy with commuter traffic. I sprinted to her; I caught her up in my arms as she planted her first foot in the gutter. When a female motorist who had anticipated the unfolding tragedy hurriedly slowed her car and cursed me, I bowed my head in shame. And as I clutched my baby daughter to my chest and returned to the house, I sobbed with equal parts guilt and gratitude.

For weeks I couldn't even confide in my wife what had happened. Even now the memory pains me to where I can't ask, what if? All I know is, I don't think I could have recovered from the loss and my responsibility in it. The loss of a child never mends, I've been told. You are never whole again. The loss to illness is one thing, but to accident—one you could have prevented—is another too horrible to live down.

Nature supplanted negligence with my second daughter Madeleine. Small from birth, she hadn't yet reached three years when my wife and I saw her fall and strike her head against the hall wall. She didn't move, seemed not to even be breathing. I watched the color leave her; she seemed to be going rigid. I rushed to call 911 while Timarie lifted the toddler's stiffening body in her arms just as my first-generation son Kurt showed up at the front door.

Memoirs of a Geezer Dad

"Kurt! Quick! Get the paramedics," I shouted.

Without a word my son sprinted the half-block to the fire station while my wife carried what appeared to be our dying daughter out onto the front lawn. I followed them, staring at the frantic mother and pallid child in a state beyond panic, having hit bottom in the abyss of angst.

It might have been a long minute before the firemen and my son arrived. Remarkably, Madeleine was already stirring, and before our relieved if confused eyes the color started returning to her face, and her limbs moved. The paramedics checked her out as her recovery and my relief continued. After five minutes they seemed satisfied they had done all they could, advising my wife and me to have a doctor check her out as soon as we could.

We did. Our pediatrician found nothing amiss, but referred us to a neurosurgeon at Children's Hospital of Orange County to play it safe. The appointment was made for two weeks off. But in a matter of days, before our scheduled appointment, Maddy had another episode. After striking her nose on the footboard of her bed, she let out one short cry, then went instantly rigid, with a leg curled underneath her. Her pallor went from gray to a faint bluish cast. Another 911 call. This time my wife and I had the paramedics take her directly to the nearest hospital's Emergency Room, my wife riding in the back of the ambulance with her, while I followed close behind in the van, but driving oh-so slowly, my limbs undulating like palsied noodles.

No sooner had I got there than our pale little girl was well on her way to the pink of recovery. Much to our puzzlement and relief, we watched her bask in the attention she got from passing nurses and attendants who commented on how cute she was. One nurse gave her a doughnut to nibble on; from Mom she got a purse to go through, allowed to open tubes of lipstick for study and application.

Fear and Trembling

"I love you, Mom," Maddy suddenly said from her emergency room cot.

"That's sweet. I love you, too," Timarie said. "What makes you say that?"

"I love you of bringing me here," the tot said, bubbling over with gratitude.

The comic relief was welcome, but did nothing for the problem we had. At least we had a lot of fresh hospital lab work—replete with MRIs and EEGs—to forward to the specialist for evaluation before our appointment.

On that nervous day, my wife and I sat twitching in Dr. Fowler's office while the learned man checked out our daughter. He didn't drag out the suspense.

"Nothing serious," he said. "Pallid Infantile Syncope."

Pallid infantile *what?*

"Please explain that in terms I can understand," demanded my wife, who is never cowed by doctors, regardless of reputation.

"Pallid infantile syncope, also known as reflex anoxic seizure or Stephenson's seizure. Unexpected pain or fright triggers a temporary cutting off of the blood supply to the brain, and the child pales, goes limp, and then faints. Usually the child recovers consciousness spontaneously in a few minutes."

How come I had never heard of such a thing? It called to mind Shakespeare's line about "the thousand natural shocks that flesh is heir to." Had he lived in our modern age of mushrooming medical knowledge, he surely would have upped the ante to a half-million.

"It's very common among toddlers," Dr. Fowler reassured my wife, whose expression showed doubt.

Very common? Maybe to this specialist, who went on to describe the condition in some detail, including the trauma-induced clenching of the jaw, stiffening of the body, jerky movement in arms and legs, then a limpness as the heart starts pumping again and the body relaxes. So accurate. Madeleine had been there, done all that.

"Nothing to worry about," he added. "She'll outgrow it."

Dr. Fowler was right. Madeleine never had another episode. And I was discovering more wisdom in the bard. Yes, there were more afflictions in heaven and earth than were dreamt of in my philosophy or described in my copy of the *Family Medical Encyclopedia*, where I was wont to browse for maladies from time to time. No more would I open the tome. Where ignorance is bliss, 'tis folly to be wise.

My choosing ignorance had no effect at all on my fear and trembling, which Madeleine unwittingly perpetuated as my regular contact point with the hospitals of Orange County. The brave little red-headed girl who liked to say "I'm big" took us through a double inguinal hernia operation, a couple gymnastic injuries, and a broken leg.

Curiously, I had never known a broken bone with my first three sons, all of whom were very physical, even hyperactive. It took my two girls to accomplish that with some seemingly harmless living-room horseplay. While wrestling, the younger, slighter Madeleine pulled her older sister back until she fell on top of her. The little one's screams began immediately and continued. My wife and I looked to one another. This wasn't just another brawl bruise.

A rushed call to 911 brought our paramedic friends from the nearby fire station again, and after what seemed too long a delay, it was off to the ER, where a spiral break of the tibia was found, later the bone set, and then a petite pink cast wrapped around my daughter's lower left leg.

Our new invalid brought me out of piggybacking retirement for three weeks as I toted the little featherweight around the house on my back. The attendant huffing and puffing confirmed there was a difference between being a parent now and the first time I tried it with young lungs and sound knees. Another thing had changed besides my physical condition. The paramedics' conduct when they first answered our distress call should have tipped me off right away. Though we were certainly not on intimate terms, they were familiar with our address, and their politely cool behavior when they first arrived was somewhat confounding. They insisted on getting a detailed version of the accident from each family member. Initially I was puzzled, then quickly grew increasingly irritated; my daughter was wailing with pain and needed attention—now! What in the world was going on?

Came the slow dawn....They were sleuthing for signs of child abuse, a new responsibility society had placed on their broad but inexperienced shoulders, forced now to peer into the dark closet of family secrets that stayed closed during my first stint as a parent. That explained their almost standoffish behavior.

I myself had entered this dangerous new reality a few years earlier. It was a Sunday and I was preparing to drive to the nearby recycling center to drop off old newspapers when three-year-old Madeleine fell from her wagon and began crying. To soothe her I offered a ride with Daddy. She still had tears in her eyes when I released the van's back door and a trio of workers— two men and a woman—began unloading the bundles of paper.

"Why are you crying?" the woman solicitously asked my daughter through the side window.

"Because my Dad hits me all the time," said Madeleine.

The woman froze, frowned, and said nothing. Her two companions, having tossed the last bundles into the dumpster, suddenly turned their heads toward me. Stunned into silence, I stared blank-faced at the three of them, powerless to defend myself against the monstrous libel. Who would believe me anyway over a sweet little charmer with tears in her eyes? Before anyone could think of anything to say, I hit the ignition and blasted off in the van, my absolute innocence put all the more in doubt, no doubt. I had to question my survival chances in this brave new world.

Just because I show ultimate concern about the health of my children does not mean I'm very good at caring for their health needs. In fact, I give myself rather low marks as a nurse. It's

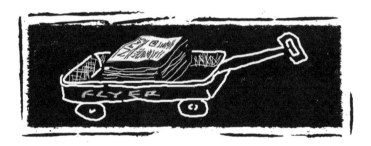

about my bedside manner. You might call it brusque, but I call it the tough-love medical approach. When dutifully spooning out palliatives, I like to bark out gruff orders to the patient to "get well soon." If only my failings ended there. They don't.

My wife has taken CPR courses offered by all manner of good folks and local organizations and has long lobbied me to do the same. "It gives you such relief to know what to do in an emergency," she repeatedly assures me.

I believe her. And I keep promising her I will. But I never get around to it. Why? That's a nettlesome question that rubs raw some deep-seated personal weaknesses rooted in irrational fears that force the pursuant trembling. Isn't to prepare for an accident an invitation to fate to bring it on? And what if I botched the rescue job? I suppose it's a variation on the family habit of avoiding doctors because it's their business to find something wrong with you. No go, no trouble.

Fear and Trembling

By way of mitigation, I did watch my wife pop a wad of ham out of Franz's windpipe with the Heimlich hold once. I'm reasonably confident I could manage the maneuver in a time of critical need, at the cost of no more than a broken rib or two. I'm not a total loser.

Close behind my fear that one of the children will face a life-or-death situation with only me to save them is that some day my bypassed heart will quit while I am home alone with my minor children. They would be under the pressure of calling 911, then perhaps watch me expire before their very eyes, before help came in time. Any scenario I could conjure would scar them for life…perhaps saddle them with the guilt that they did wrong or somehow could have done more.

Three-and-a-half years after the surgery, fear-of became might-be. It was 6:33 p.m. of a Friday evening, my wife working late, and I was putting hamburger buns in the oven for warming when the world turned upside down. Or my head did. I caught myself against a counter and staggered into the living room and my La-Z-Boy near the phone. There, supine, the spinning world accelerated, and I felt the rush of nausea attended by a horrendous sweat.

"Molly," I gasped, "call 911. Hurry!"

"What's wrong?" asked the alarmed girl just-turned 13, whom I had always feared would panic in just such circumstances.

"Dizzy. Can't stand. Call for help—now!"

With aplomb she did just that, and had the sense to mention that I had had heart surgery.

Molly later said the paramedics arrived in just five minutes, though it seemed longer to a guy who felt trapped inside a

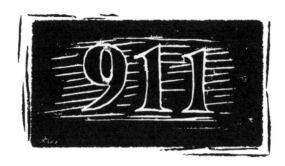

turning kaleidoscope and who greeted them with the first spume of vomit.

The team of six went right to work, treating me for a heart attack even as they questioned me. I laboriously gave them curt answers between the barfings:

Age? "Sixty-six." (They kept asking my birth date.... I kept wanting to move it forward to give myself a better chance.)

Hospital of choice? "Hoag."

Chest pains? "Didn't feel like it."

From the onset I deep-down doubted my heart was at fault, and as the gurney was lifted into the ambulance I told a medic, "I might have food poisoning." If so, my surviving heirs would benefit from a handsome settlement from a well-known national pizza merchant whose fare I had just consumed. My confidence flagged, though, when I overheard an attendant give my blood pressure—188 over 140—to a buddy. That high pressure wasn't like me at all!

"Can you help us get your tee-shirt off?" the medic asked me. I couldn't. Couldn't move my body that much. Besides, a flood of perspiration had literally bonded the cotton to my skin. So, in the few calms between the puking episodes, the paramedics cut the shirt off of me.

Then I remembered...the buns in the oven. Not a Second Act house fire! Through gasps I prevailed on an attendant to use his cell phone to call Molly and have her turn the oven off. The nausea intensified, and I had to conclude that the end was near. Which seemed preferable to a continuing life distinguished only by torrents of sweat and barf.

An odd mix the last thoughts I had…satisfaction that my life insurance premiums were paid up, frustration that my "Geezer Dad" manuscript would never be completed, regrets that I hadn't told my wife not to have me cremated, so I wouldn't be entropy's agent and hasten the depletion of the universe's supply of energy.

I remember stop-and-go fragments of my transfer from ambulance to emergency room to the cardiac ward. I remember my wife was there, putting up a brave front and joking with doctors and staff. Early assurances that my heart was not at fault relieved my wife but were lost on me. All I wanted was an end to the paroxysms that shook my body.

Only the next morning, 14 hours after my dizziness began, did I hear the comforting words from a bright young neurosurgeon that I was in no danger. Preliminary diagnosis? Probably benign vertigo, triggered by a viral infection of the inner ear. *Vertigo?* Yes, what I thought was merely a conceit of Alfred Hitchcock turned out to be another of those "fairly common conditions" that I now shared with the multitudes. Of course, an MRI would be necessary to confirm that something more serious wasn't the cause. A tortuous procedure for us poor claustrophobes who can't stand the boiler-room banging and clanking while strapped into a torpedo tube, but I had undergone one before and would again to verify the diagnosis. Done, even before my body started returning to firm ground with the aid of Antivert.

Memoirs of a Geezer Dad

Geezer fathers scan dark clouds for silver linings. I found one in the groundless fear that Molly would panic, become hysterical, if I should brush death's door before her eyes. Not so. She had proved a cool heroine under fire, a stalwart chip off the matriarchal block, so much better prepared now to handle life's future, often trying, surprises.

Maybe I can persuade her to take CPR.

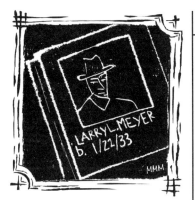

Chapter 17

Existential
Living

*A*S EVERY GARDEN variety existentialist knows, the central fact of life is death. Yes, for us, existence does indeed precede essence. Yes, our awareness of our mortality sets up a tension that leads to anguish, abandonment, and despair—until the self asserts its will and decides to choose and become an individual human unlike all others…or fails to do so in that short span of years we have to be.

No surprise then that my age and circumstances provide the existential bedrock of our family life. Death, and the sorrow and disruption it brings to a family, can't be shunted off to some vague future 30 or 40 years off. It is a fact of everyday life, as real as the blood pressure medicine the kids see me take every day. And for this life-long thanatophobe, death lurks as a daily possibility, an uneasy presence that tells me my time with those I love could end today with the sudden bursting of an artery wall.

So I live a double life. The public one is as the time-on-his-hands retiree husband to a young wife and father of young children—a regular at Girl Scout bridging ceremonies and Cub Scout pack meetings, wearing a smile over shaky knees and achy hips. The second life, the buried life, belongs to an old man with a compulsion to check daily the obituary page for friends and acquaintances just departed. We—those noted on the newspaper pages as well as those waiting to go—belong to the "Mar-Mar" generation, consumers of martinis and

Memoirs of a Geezer Dad

Marlboros, for whom the Surgeon General's warning came too late. We have paid the price in reduced longevity. Lung cancer, bone cancer, congestive heart failure have taken my three closest friends, and I have written their obituaries. It's a grim business I choose not to share with my family. Keep the mourning to myself…let the buoyancy of young life rise undamped.

The die-off of my generation peaked last year. In one week I read obits for a friend and a close acquaintance—both taken before age 65 by the Big C. The friend was Tom, the sometime writer, sometime editor, all-the-time idealist who offered me my first book contract. We drank too much gin together and laughed too hard. That had to be paid for. He was a man whose first love was the wilderness, the defense of which he made his life's work. Noble work, well done.

The acquaintance I'd scraped fangs with several times in the political snake pit known as Academic Life. I thought her self-important and humorless in the days we served on committees together. But now I can only think of what a devoted teacher of literature she was, and the high standards she set for her students, and how she was a force for good in the world while she lived. Odd how we are bound to members of our own generation by shared experiences—including conflict.

These roster cuts keep me active pulling and chucking cards from my Rolodex and taping clipped obits into my journal on the proper death day. I always pen in a few lines of personal farewell—a well-meaning but feeble attempt to honor and remember old mates. Probably no one ever will read these words…or know my feelings for that dead friend…which is itself another death of a sort…verbal remains piled on already moldering corpses in the graveyard of memory.

My wife senses when I'm in one of my mortality funks. "You've got to get out more," she says. "You should see your friends."

Existential Living

"They're all dead," I'm apt to snap. They're not, of course. When I slip out to a funeral or wake I see old friends among fellow mourners. We will shake hands or embrace and laugh and remember and take each other's new addresses and phone numbers and promise to stay in touch. But we don't. Why? Because the way we were is never the way we are. What bound our lives in time and place has been severed. Their interests have changed with their new lifestyles—to golf and tennis and travel and volunteer work. Most have moved farther out of town and can't hack long freeway drives; many are not wired and never will have e-mail addresses.

"Why don't you *phone* Frances?" my ever-solicitous wife will suggest after I've spoken nostalgically of a dear old friend.

I would like to but I won't. I lack the courage to intrude on fellow survivors grappling with their own infirmities. Whatever ideas we might have to share soon give way to the inevitable kvetch sessions in which we compare states of decay and complain about which digestive organ is not pulling its weight, or which over-rated painkiller gives no relief at all.

Or worse, as has happened to me once, you phone your fellow survivor only to divine in the strained conversation that lamely follows that he is not well. He is in fact terminal. Imminently so. And you must say your brief farewells without rehearsal, on the spot. Those are the times that try the soul.

"Have you thought of making new friends?" my wife asks, ever mindful of my moods.

Easier said than done. Age militates against forming new friendships. There is that requisite community of interests, rooted in shared experiences, to begin with. And where would I go to find it? Take Frost's road not taken and wend my way to Leisure World, where seniors my age flock to face the coming extinction bravely and together? Join the other tourists leisurely heading home?

Memoirs of a Geezer Dad

While I envy them their peace of mind and sense of completion, I think not. Golf reveals the vilest side of my personality. Bridge exposes me as a memory-challenged dunderhead. And dance the hula at the monthly luau? Not this prime candidate for double hip replacement!

Nor, do I suspect, would I be welcomed by those smiling tanned seniors sipping Chardonnay in the clubhouse. There's the baggage I bring, including the wife and kids. How could I explain to them why a doddering old man would want to go through parenting a second time? Endure the impossible rigors of being a good father again when you've already put two-plus decades into the job and are still hoping you did it right? That's the kind of pain-freak you don't want to hang out with in your golden years.

No, I am no mellow senior, nor was meant to be. I confess to the same grand weakness Camus's man Jean-Baptiste Clamence admitted to: I love life too much—so much that I'm incapable of imagining what is not life. I want to be with the young and the younger, since it is they who seem to have a monopoly on living, even if they don't make the most of it. I think I do and choose to be a straggler as my generation exits; I mean to mingle with those who follow…associate with young people doing young things—even though I may be a rather passive participant. It sure beats the alternative.

Two decades-plus ago a dirty old reprobate pal told me the secret to his long life was breathing the breath of a young woman. I have followed that advice for the last 20 years, extending my time among the quick beyond what I've otherwise earned.

I might now applaud myself for the choice I made, but the credit goes to my wife Timarie, my former student 27 years my junior, the love of my life who accepted me. A couple's song says it all. Ours is "Younger Than Springtime" from *South

Existential Living

Pacific. I call her Springtime because she is my Liat, my well-spring of laughter and optimism who gave me reasons to live when I first met her and gives many more to continue now. Which brings us to crux time and, I suppose, the real reason for this lengthy document.

No surprise that as our April-October match has matured into a July-December union, tears are sometimes shed…nobody stiffs the piper. At least twice a year, usually at night in bed a major lamentation session overtakes us, during which we review and then sanction the choices we've made.

Never are these intense nights planned, but rather are reactive to some happening in the course of living the day. Typical was the night we watched the film *Shadowlands* together. The moving story of C. S. Lewis losing to cancer the youngish woman he loved blindsided us, drove home the transient nature of our own bond, freed the wash of tears that brought our own reality back into sharp focus. Similar evenings have followed, amounting almost to rites of intensification, in which we discuss necessary plans that must be uncomfortably made. When I fret over my guilt for leaving her and the kids in a bad way, she reminds me that *she* made a conscious choice to have a family with me, knowing the time together would be briefer than most. We agree that my passing will be hardest for her to bear. It's easier to die. It's much harder to live on as a survivor, particularly given that the females of her line live long, and she may face 40-plus years of living alone. Find a good man to share them with, I tell her. Life belongs to the living.

We conclude every session thankful that we have had 20 fine years with one another and agreed that whatever is left is a gift not to be wasted. We vow to squeeze it of every joyful possibility, to make our sun run by seizing every day, gathering every rosebud while we may.

For me, this is a new way of living that Timarie (abetted by the aging process) has had to teach me. Most of my past life I spent worrying about the future or regretting my past, with the present a negligible bridge between the two. Now, with so little future out there to plan for, and so much past to even try to remember, I live in the eternal present, stretch time as best I can. Shelved are the selfish thoughts that I was marked for greater things that must necessarily distance me from those I live with each day. Slowly, and perhaps naturally, I have come to treasure Saturday's soccer mornings with my kids in their queer-looking togs, the gym-sweat-scented evenings spent watching a daughter's slow elfin mastery of the parallel bars, the seasonal performances of a ten-year-old supernumerary in a *Nutcracker* matinee.... These are the real stuff of life. Live for now and banish rancor—that's my version of living well as the best revenge. It sure beats past paths I've trod.

The path I now walk is blessed with children just getting their first look at the world and its tawdry wonders, a welcome tonic for my hard-earned cynicism. I love to talk to them, on any subject, on any pretext. I find myself dragging our conversations out, wanting to absorb their fresh ideas and to teach them what I know of life and point them toward my values. But most of all I indulge myself with love cloaked in words.

Death occasionally worms its way into those conversations, with my death always a swollen subtext. I try to be unemotional about the subject, spout in a rational voice all that death-is-a-natural-rounding-out-of-life rot. How well it soothes them I'm not sure. I do know that all my kids are chips off the existential block and became aware of their mortality early—and don't like it at all. Usually the discovery comes between the age of three and four and is accompanied by that all-important human change we call self-awareness. For a long time my oldest son Eric held the record of first crossing the threshold to being. He had just turned three when he followed me into my bedroom one day and announced, with tears in his eyes, "I don't want to die."

"I know," I said. "But you have to."

Some bedside manner! Sad to say, it hasn't improved in 34 years. I still don't know how to soften the blow.

We were driving in the van when Franz, at age two years, six months and 13 days, eclipsed Eric's record by asking me and the world at large from his infant seat: "Do we have to die?"

"Yes, I'm afraid we do," I said.

His fair face clouded over. The purblind doomsters had busted into another life announcing man's fate. My heart ached for him, my final child, this accidental son whose coming I had dreaded, but who now had become my boon buddy who gives a special luster to each day.

Exactly a week later after I confirmed the bad news. Again in the van and traveling to his baby sitter's, Franz asked, "Dad, when are you going to die?"

"I don't know," I responded in a detached voice. It was a ready defense I would find convenient on future occasions.

Madeleine, my five-year-old kindergartner hurried to the rescue: "In a thousand million thirty weeks—that's a long time."

I liked her answer, but wanted it put in writing...and she couldn't write. I could and I would. Then and there I resolved to write down in my journal future conversations on the subject—lessen its sting the way John Donne did in his sonnets, cutting death down to size with the magic of words. Not that it would prolong our life together. But it would leave a record, for Franz or anyone interested in a seat-of-the-pants, non-scientific "clinical" study of how a child copes with the idea of a parent's death...and, indirectly I suppose, how a geezer father prepares himself for the last goodbye.

What follows is a brief abstract of those conversations, mostly with my youngest son, over the last eight years. My daughters, too, have such concerns, but they are older and tend to confide them in my wife, and in any case are much more tactful than my son, who is all boy, wide open, what you hear is what he is. I've selected these particular scenes from an existential family life to try to show a pattern in a clumsy coming to terms with the inevitable.

5/20/95. Franz at two years, eight months, and 23 days awakens me at 3:30 a.m. with the patter of his sleeper feet coming down the hall toward the master bedroom. I hear him crying. I get up and throw open the door, and he rushes past me into his mother's arms.

"What's wrong?" my wife asks.

"I thought my dad was lost," he sobs.

A knife cut through my heart. Guilt commingled with sorrow as I realized that the prospect of life without me for him was as terrifying as life without him was to me. The emotional moment drove home the duty I had to last as long as I could, try to reach the time when he could survive the loss of his father without lasting damage to the person he would become. As for me, not to have this child to love and watch grow each day would be life void of joy.

9/25/96. Adjustments came in time. Two days before his fourth birthday, Franz looked into my face and asked, "Are you old?"

"Yes, I'm old," I said, choosing flat-out honesty over all the possible hedges.

He thought a few seconds, apparently reviewing what he knew of dying and how it related to age, then cut me some slack: "But not too old."

"No, not too old," I hastily agreed. I was on my sixth day of taking DHEA and feeling better already.

10/25/96. Exactly a month later, as I sat in my La-Z-Boy, he was back to confront me with a question that suggested he'd been plumbing my medical history. "Are your lungs still black from smoking?" he asked.

"No, I quit smoking 18 years ago. They're pink again."

His gaze steadied. He seemed satisfied. I liked the idea that he was on the case. Just so he didn't join his sister Molly in nagging me about the cholesterol in my diet.

1/20/97. Apparently I had a morning appointment 11 weeks later because he was back with a prognosis, delivered very matter-of-factly: "Dad, you're going to die soon."

I sat frozen in my chair. Had the kid been consulting my cardiologist behind my back? "How do you know?"

"Because you have gray hair."

I felt somewhat relieved. There was always Grecian Formula to buy me some time. "There are a lot of men with gray hair walking around, very much alive," I told him.

"They will be dead soon," he assured me.

Soon? Well, why press the issue. All the same, this new clinical (or should I say "callous"?) turn of mind I found vaguely unsettling at first. The boy was seeing life and death in simple black and white, without color, apparently death without tears. But then again, isn't that what I wanted? Or at least a move in that direction of acceptance, away from excess grief? Couldn't hurt.

I found myself picking up on his brave new approach to my demise by speaking about it openly when appropriate. Kind of getting the family used to the idea of a time when I wouldn't be around, and perhaps appealing at the same time to whatever caring gods there be that I not be taken before I'd met my obligations. Letting the kids know I didn't intend to go gentle into that good night.

Less than a month after getting the death sentence for my gray hair I told my wife casually at the dinner table that, "if I

live to my next birthday," I looked forward to her baking the butter almond cake she had recently mastered.

The table erupted with words. Not my favorite? Not the
pineapple upside down cake that my mother used to bake and
Timarie had often simulated for the birthdays past? Did I really
want to switch?

Franz seemed to be listening to the blather, but quickly interrupted to turn the conversation elsewhere, namely to himself,
specifically to whether he could play both professional baseball
and professional basketball when he grew up.

Never wanting to hobble ambition, I told him "yes," it was
possible, scratching memory for someone besides Gene Conley.

"And I can play football, too," he exclaimed, delighted that
his imagined abilities would not be thwarted by rules of any kind.

I was just about to explain how overlapping seasons pretty
much prevented one from playing all three major sports professionally when Madeleine, who had heard me speak slightingly of
football and warn of the possibility of early injury, piped up:

"No you can't. Dad won't let you."

Even as Madeleine looked to me for confirmation of the judgment, Franz fired a ready rejoinder: "He'll be dead by then," he
said with unruffled certainty.

The table grew silent. I started to stammer a "not-so-fast"
protest. Instead an image moved front and center into my mind.
It was of little John John, brave and tearless, making a soldierly
salute to his father's casket on that cold November day so long
ago. Hard facts and quick action sweep away personal tears and
static mourning for little boys. Thank God for little boys.

Too soon Franz moved from the fearless fives to the scholas-
tic sixes where I became a convenient math-learning aid. He

became fascinated with punching my age into a calculator, then adding a single digit number and announcing to me how old I would be in x more years. I had to congratulate him on his newfound competence with figures. But I wished he'd get done with the sums and move on to the take-aways.

Instead math somehow got enmeshed with history as the boy approached age seven. Example? We were watching a baseball game together, as is our wont, and Vin Scully was discussing Joe Dimaggio's 1941 streak of hitting in 56 straight games and Ted Williams hitting above .400, when Franz asked me, "How old were you when that happened?"

"Eight."

"How old were you in 1949?"

"Sixteen."

"How old were you in 1956?"

"Twenty-three. It was the year I got out of the Air Force." I had hoped this might deflect him, and I could sidetrack him with some war stories.

"How old were you in 1965?

"Thirty-two. That's the year your brother Eric was born." He didn't take the bait.

"How old were you in 1983?"

"Fifty. Now let's watch the Dodger game."

We had finally moved on to subtraction, but I was doing all the work, and I didn't much care for my life serving as his personal abacus.

Franz's obsession with my age continued, the lad's rational and indirect way of handling my end creeping into the details of daily living and touching me always. Take my last day in Academia. Following my retirement from full-time teaching, I did sign on to teach history and literature part-time at one of those multi-branched universities catering to working adults. Though the classroom give-and-take was as usual mentally exhilarating and great for slowing down the geezering process, meddling classroom flops promoted to administrative positions made the job miserable, and I ended my teaching career at age 65 on a sour note.

My last act within the ivyless walls—once the last student had turned in his final exam for Great World Literature and left—was to go to the blackboard and chalk in big and bold letters, "William Butler Yeats is the greatest!" I knew the janitors would likely erase this weird manifesto before any of the staff saw it and puzzled over its meaning.

When I got home I told my family at the dinner table of my last obscure act of defiance.

"Who was William Butler Yeats?" my future scholar daughter Molly asked.

"The greatest poet of our time," I said. "Maybe all time."

"Is he dead?" Molly asked.

"Yes," I said.

"What did he die of?" Madeleine asked.

"Of old age," my wife said, giving what has become our stock answer. "He was lucky. He died an old, old man."

Franz, who had been a silent listener through it all, got up from his chair, came over and hugged me. "My Dad is going to be lucky," he said, coming of age.

I felt a rush of love and a swelling in my throat along with a warm reassurance. If only wishing made it so.

In six months' time the boy, probably beset by fresh doubts, caught me alone for some background information. "How old was your father?"

"You mean when he died?"

"Yes."

"Seventy-eight."

"How old was your mother."

"Sixty-five," I said reluctantly.

He wrinkled his brow, but said nothing. Was the young dinosaur-scientist-to-be with a flair for math going to interpolate? Maybe, better, extrapolate? How much time did he think I had, and how would that influence how we spent out our final days together?

These preoccupations with our coming separation continued to dog our days together. If a person's name was mentioned casually, he would ask, "Is he (she) alive?"

I would say "yes," to which there was no response, or "no," which brought the usual question, "What did he die of?"

"I don't know...bad heart, I think." (Or some variation thereon.)

"How old was he?" is the almost inevitable follow-up.

I always hope we're discussing an octogenarian, and I tend to fudge my answers in that direction, as in "somewhere in his eighties."

"And you're only in your sixties?"

"Yes." We never mention that it's the high-sixties. How nice to get his support, though.

Franz took a major step toward acceptance when he reached age eight and a half.

"You know why *Charlotte's Web* is a good story, Dad?" he asked me. (His mother had just finished reading him the E. B. White classic.)

"Why is that?"

"Because Charlotte teaches Wilbur things you have to know, and then Charlotte dies, and then Wilbur teaches those things to her children. That's the way it should be, isn't it, Dad?"

"Yes," I said, without elaborating on those valuable lessons of death and survival and continuity. It was becoming clear to me that I was the follower and he would lead me to where we had to go.

Memoirs of a Geezer Dad

That happened on tax day 2002 as I drove him home from baseball practice.

"Do you ever wonder what dying will be like?" he asked me from out of nowhere.

"As a matter of fact, I do, from time to time."

"Me, too." He paused. "I don't want you to die," he added in a thick voice.

"I don't want to, either," I said, fending off a quaver.

"Dad, when you die, how will I get to school?"

"Maybe you'll be driving by then…at least I hope so."

A two-second pause. "And I don't want a step-dad, either," he said through puffy lips.

Bless the boy! Education a top priority! And he thinks his Dad is irreplaceable! As for those future living arrangements, he'd have to work those out with his mother.

Ten days later he hoisted the practical to the sublime. We were alone again in the van on our way home from school when he said, "Life is very fragile. When it breaks, we are gone."

"Those are beautiful words," I said, stunned that they were obviously his alone.

"The earth is a shelf and we are vases. When one vase falls and breaks, all of them get chipped."

What a metaphor! Meet your nine-year-old match, Mr. Donne!

The above entries are interspersed, indeed merge, with theological topics discussed even less conclusively, as in, "Dad, why did God make pitbulls?"

"I don't know." (And I don't.)

"Dad, is heaven higher than the world?"

"That's what they say." (A cheap cop-out, sure, but how am

I to know whether he means geographically higher or a loftier state of being?)

"Dad, can God bite through a dinosaur's neck?"

"I suppose so...if God chooses to." (How deftly Dad side-steps the gender trap by avoiding the divine pronoun.) "But why would God want to bite the neck of a dinosaur?"

Franz brushes aside the question as irrelevant, goes on to his own: "Why did God make dinosaurs?"

"Same reason for making pitbulls, I guess...carnivores keep down animal over-populations." My voice is unconvincing, because it's a variation on the old God-authoring-evil conundrum with overtones of the nature-red-in-tooth-and-claw enigma, neither of which I can reconcile. "Hey buddy! Why don't you get the bat and whiffle ball, and I'll pitch you a few?"

"Wait! I'll get the bat!" It worked! Questions vaporize. He can't believe the old arthritic has agreed to throw his back out again.

These artful dodges stem from my respect for religious faith and my resolve not to tamper with what is a gift that gives life meaning and purpose. At the same time, faith can't be willed...at least by me. As the issue of a German Catholic mother and a German Lutheran father, schooled in a university English department with a strong Calvinist bent, addicted to reading *Scientific American* (admittedly, only a third of which I understand), I see at least four sides to every question and come by my skepticism naturally enough. My life-long pilgrimage for spiritual meaning has left me both a cultural Catholic and a default deist with teleological leanings suspect in a universe apparently condemned to expand forever.

My Roman Catholic wife, on the other hand, is gifted with faith, and when that wavers, I have noticed, hope successfully rushes in to the rescue. The both of us are committed to raising our children Catholic, which makes me a cautious and inadequate source of religious truth. No, I can't give the kids those yes or no answers right on the spot. I am myself a seeker of truth still, doomed to never know the answers to their questions and many more of my own—answers, I suspect, more bewilderingly beautiful and wonderful than I have the capacity to imagine.

Stuck in my mind is a scenario Franz, age five, fashioned for us on February 21, 1997, at the breakfast table.

"Dad, when I go to heaven, I'll be an angel. You'll already be an angel, too. Isn't that right?"

"That's what they say."

"That'll be great! Dad, we'll be able to fly!"

His words stir deep yearnings in my hardened heart's core. I choke off an imminent sob with a self-administered apothegm: With a trillion galaxies each hosting 100 billion or so stars, it would seem that all things possible are in fact inevitable.

Would I ever like to fly as his wingman! We might just go out and catch a falling star!

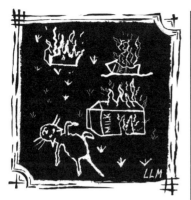

Chapter 18

My Advice
to You

hAVING SPENT MOST of my life in journalism, or teaching
that dubious subject, I reluctantly add to this self-indulgent memoir (meant mainly as a memento for my kids) a chapter of practical advice. After all, why not pay this age of so-
called service journalism its due? Give you something useful for
your money? And maybe boost book sales with some tried-and-
true "how to" advice under the teaser line, "My Ten Top Tips
on Child Rearing."

You might rightly ask, "Is this guy really qualified to give
advice?" To which I glibly reply that none of my six children is
presently doing time, and all six are paying taxes. Another
qualification is that—in defiance of my wife's wishes—I've
never read a book on parenting. Why? Probably for the same
reason I don't ask for directions when I get lost on Southern
California's meandering streets. Again, why? I don't know and
don't want to know. But I do know I wouldn't have the time
for those books anyway after doing the day's required reading—
the sports page, the front page, the editorial page, the book
reviews, the obits, not to mention the six magazines I subscribe
to and fail to read to my money's worth.

My beet-faced uncle Otto used to cock his bald head and say
to me through the teeth clenched around his pipe, "Too zoon
vee get oldt; too late vee get schmardt." I know I've gotten old.
I like to think I've gotten smarter and have learned through six
separate trials and many more errors how to make being a father

somewhat easier. (Dare I pretend to success as well?) Put another way, my advice is intuitive, rooted in the experience of trying to raise six quite different children as a mainstream American pragmatist ultimately committed to "whatever works." So here goes.

1. Let Them Be

The hardest lesson I learned as a father is that your children are not replicates of yourself—despite the DNA you supplied. They are all different, ones of a kind. Having subscribed to nature over nurture even before Crick and Watson exposed the double helix, I viewed my first three sons as extensions of their father. Thus defined, I would shape them to fit the futures I had chosen for them. As I mentioned earlier, I meant to guide Eric of the argumentative ways into being a counterculture lawyer serving the down-and-out deadbeats he admired from the day of his birth. (He's now the general contractor.) Kurt the slick jock would hit for power and average in the three slot for a Major League baseball team—preferably the Dodgers. (He now teaches community college English literature.) Karl the musical-minded would perform Rodrigo's guitar concerti in the world's premier concert halls. (He owns a sculpture studio catering to the entertainment industry.) That's zero for three in the parental molding league.

Worse was the outright defiance I got for my pains. It seemed the harder I tried to push them in a direction I thought was good for them, the more they dug in their heels and went another. I remember the day when the extent of their rebellion peaked, and even I couldn't help but see it for what it was. Eric at age 12 came up to me and asked, somewhat belligerently I thought, "Dad, do you know what my favorite sport is?"

He knew my preferences—baseball, basketball and football, team sports I had pushed him and his brothers into, as befitted one of my urban, proletarian background. So maybe he'd chosen tennis.... Okay for a child of the rebellious, individualistic Sixties.

"Moto-Cross."

Moto-Cross! That idiotic time-waste for juvenile delinquents he had heard me rail against for years. The smile on his face bordered on a sneer as he punctured my elitist balloon and declared his absolute independence from me and all my future plans for him.

It was a lesson well-learned. For my second family I have backed off and given my children the space to be themselves. Of course that led to problems as well. Once you concede that children are all different, and one size does not fit all, then logic dictates that rules governing their conduct must be flexible as well. Yes, bending rules sets a dangerous precedent, as most parents know. But I find myself doing it anyway—and learning new child-rearing strategies in the process.

Take the case of Madeleine entering the first grade. She attended the first two days, then caught a sniffle and missed the third. It cleared up quickly and she was fine to return on the fourth.

"I'm sick. I'm not going to school," she cried when awakened in the morning.

Now I was raised in the "Malingerers Beware!" tradition of parenthood. Kid, you better not be faking it! Because if you're too sick to go to school, then you're too sick to watch television, and you're too sick to go out and play once school's out. That was my father's rule, and it became mine. Rigid. No flex to it.

215

Memoirs of a Geezer Dad

"You'll have to go school, Maddy," I said, maybe a bit too firmly. "Don't worry. You'll be fine."

"No, I won't go."

"Look, being with other kids will be good for you," I said in a lapse of logic.

"I won't go." Her resolve was hardening, and I could sense that it already exceeded that of Eric the Stubborn.

I was about to bluster and go to my "Oh-yes-you-will" command when emotions—my emotions—intervened. "Come here, and let me hold you," I found myself suddenly blurting instead.

She stiffened momentarily, then rushed into my arms. I sat and rocked her for 20 seconds or so. "You're scared, aren't you?"

Her lips quivered in a prelude to denial.

"I understand. You missed a day, and you think they won't remember you. They will. They love you, Maddy. Everybody loves you."

She gave in…well, part way. "Can I take some marshmallows to school?" asked the constant conner, always two maneuvers ahead of me.

"You know they have snacks at school. You don't want to take what other kids won't have," I reminded her, though both of us knew that is precisely what she wanted. Then, in an inspired moment, I said, "but we can put some in a baggie and you can eat them on the way to school."

Mollified but not quite satisfied. "I want to take my cup to school."

"Your drinking cup?" I asked, puzzled. Oh, I got it. A possession to take and show off. But strictly forbidden by school rules.

"You know we aren't allowed to do that," I said, but hurried out the Plan B compromise: "What we can do is fill it with appie (apple juice) and you can drink it on the way."

Stymied and fresh out of demands, she grudgingly gave in. Her academic career would continue.

I felt proud of my new-found flexibility, which came with an appreciation for negotiation. How far from the dogmatic patriarch I used to be.

2. Be Their Biggest Booster

If you can't make your children what *you* want them to be, why not help them become what *they* want to be? That's the logical corollary to my choice to not choose for them. Instead, I've tried to become an enabler who encourages them in all things good and neutral. (I won't encourage them if they have a penchant for bomb-building, of course.)

Go for it! You can do it! Great idea! All are standard goads I apply when they tell me of their latest plans for the future. Such cheerleading may sound like pure treacle, but it sure beats what I have observed in some parents who seem to delight in dashing their children's hopes, putting them down when they get uppity with their ambitions. It seems to me a perverse kind of envy that has them hoping their children won't become more than they were…or are. Such a pity.

Of course, I know some of the dream deflators are unaware of their actions and the stifling effect they have on those they love. Often as not it's a stolid dad, bruised badly by unfulfilling labor in the workaday world, feeling uncomfortable in the presence of a creative child prone to fantasy. The temptation to prick balloons comes naturally. But rather than lowering the boom of grim reality, I ask, Why not stay silent and listen to the bubbling of youthful imagination? It may even remind you of good times past when you thought the world your playground.

I confess that I may carry tolerance and the cheerleading too far—been too supportive of my children's every whim and dream. That was suggested by a conversation with my son

Memoirs of a Geezer Dad

Franz who came to me after playing well in an Upward League basketball game for eight-year-olds.

"Dad, do you think I'll break Michael Jordan's record?"

The question, sincerely asked, took my breath away. Talk about confidence unchecked! He had already projected himself into NBA stardom and put himself at the pinnacle of athletic fame. Was there a way to talk him down without damaging his self-esteem?

"Son, Michael Jordan was the best basketball player ever. You're just learning the game. He's an adult. You're an eight-year-old kid."

His blue eyes sank to view his chest. Had I squelched him?

"Why don't we wait and see?" I added. "And of course try our best in the meantime." I proceeded to flesh out once again the John Wooden homily on success as doing the best you can and not paying much mind to wins and losses and records and other external recognition.

He listened, and I assumed it came across as advisory, not captious. Striking the proper balance, however, remains difficult. I find this true, too, with my daughter Madeleine, who carries into a fourth year her vow to perform autopsies. "Great idea," I say, "but remember that profession requires a good deal of math—not exactly your favorite subject." A warning warranted? Or was I just trying to steer her away from such a ghoulish line of work?

So her slicing up corpses turns out to be a fantasy...what's the loss? Isn't fantasy the fraternal twin of creativity and deserving of being nourished together?

Dullard dads, listen up. Don't tread on dreams. Some of us spin fantasies to enrich our dull and undistinguished lives and become heroes and heroines (or even villains, I suppose) in imagined parallel lives. Let us go to our graves having conquered Asia without the loss of one drop of real blood, or rid-den a son of Swaps to victory in the Kentucky Derby despite burdening the steed with 230 pounds of clumsy live weight that has never gone the classic mile and a quarter before.

Dream and let dream, I say.

3. Read to Them

Trite advice. But this is a big-time winner in so many ways. You teach your child language, our most useful tool. You give him or her that academic head start so many parents seek these days. But most of all, you build strong bonds of intimacy with your child that last over time.

I won't pass myself off as the greatest practitioner of the art. But I'm married to her. Timarie started when Molly was first born, while breastfeeding, reading aloud James Joyce's *Dubliners*, an appropriately high-brow start for my most literary child, who also happens to look like Miss Galway of 2003. Tim has continued with Madeleine and Franz, going through the best children's books, back-boned by E. B. White's brilliant trilogy. Most recently she read through the Harry Potter series to a rapt audience invited aboard the master bedroom's California king after dinner. I'm always amazed to peer in when a reading is in progress and see the children still and silent in her spell, even when the subject matter is beneath or behind them. Yes, shared words, in the beginning and in the end, if we let them, bind us, fix memories.

I'm not nearly as effective as my wife in the reading game. But I have made an effort. Fear of leaving behind a son who will not remember his father guilts me into shaking the weariness off, turning the telly off, and sitting side by side on the sofa with him, sharing Stuart's descent down the drain to retrieve Mrs. Little's ring.

Memoirs of a Geezer Dad

Unfortunately, a greater guilt impairs my ability to sustain it. I'm a writer, and as such should be writing, not reading. That pushes the reluctant scribe to the word processor. To make up for not reading much to them, however, I've become their Answer Man. They are encouraged to approach me at any time with any question on any subject. Even if I am busy, I resist brushing them off with a "can't right now" or "later" and do my best to answer their question as best I can. Yes, the free access is abused at times, to where I sometimes think I'm doing their homework assignments for them. That's when I blow the whistle and tell them to go consult a dictionary or an atlas. Or to act their age and go online to Google.

4. Reach Out and Touch Them

I once heard a learned psychologist who specialized in family relations extol the virtues of touch as a keeper of domestic peace, not to mention a promoter of family harmony. He cited the closest thing to a perfect father as a rather ordinary man he knew who never failed to reach out and touch one of his children if they so much as passed in the hall. Nothing showy or too demonstrative. Just an intimate brush…a reminding pat, perhaps…a touch of love.

The words made a lasting dent on my mind—probably because I had unconsciously proven his thesis at least partially true with my first family of three boys. Having escaped my genetic due (that peculiar Northern European heterosexual male horror of skin contact with another human being of your own gender), I loved to gently maul my three baby sons born only 15 months apart who could, and did, pass for triplets.

Actually, my first-born son didn't escape that common aversion to male skin contact. As an infant he would push me away when I tried to snuggle him—a source of confused pain for this then-new father. I felt hurt, personally rejected by my own flesh and blood; I wasn't seasoned enough as a parent to know the variability in human responses is wide and not necessarily permanent.

I made it up with the others and with much horseplay, including pony rides with all three of them clinging to my back as I cantered over the carpet on sturdy palms and knees. Wrestling with all three simultaneously—rug romps that featured much huffing with squeals and howls thrown in—gave me my tactile fix and let them relieve any pent-up resentments with sharp blows to Dad's ribs. Hugs and kisses were a closing act for at least two of them.

That all changed at puberty. Touch became a casualty of their move toward independence. Most American boys feel the pressure to avoid physical contact with their peers as well as their parents, unless they are wearing football or basketball uniforms, when it is allowed—even encouraged, as long as it is violent or assertive. My sons were no exceptions. Physical contact between us sharply tapered off as they strayed into their teens. Presumably, they sought out other skin for comfort…girls their age it would seem in retrospect.

Only later, when they had grown to manhood and beyond, did we make contact again—this time with firm *abrazos*, ritualized to be sure, but laden with true affection. These are now *de rigueur* when we meet or part.

As a second-generation father blessed with two daughters, I got my second chance at child-cuddling. I also took the opportunity to test further the professor's claim about the soothing powers of touch. It worked! I would see an argument coming and go pat a head or massage a back and, presto!—the hostility would subside. Alas, again adolescence came upon the scene toting the oldest taboo that is fast-reducing my contact with my daughters to a few cheek pecks or brief pats and strokes to the bald-spot zone.

Not yet, however, with my last child and last son, the cuddliest kid of them all. From his first days as a newborn, Franz thrived on strokes. Back scratches, scalp rubs, whatever—he takes his tactile pleasure wherever and from whomever he can. He's a very trusting child, and I've wondered if trust and touch aren't boon companions.

How much more touch time with him do I have? Will adolescence bring change again? I can't predict, but I won't be the first to put my hands in my pocket.

5. Cultivate Courtesy

My wife installed this family operating system gradually and with stealth, so it was on us, in us, before we could mount much resistance. It began with such gambits as her saying, "Molly, I appreciate your hanging up your wet towel in the bathroom" and to me, "Thank you for making our lunches and dinners every day as you do." You might think I'd warm immediately to such expressions of appreciation. Nope. I grunted with resistance at first, mockingly murmuring under my breath, "And thanks for breathing, Molly," and out of her hearing to my son, "Franz, please get up and dress for school before I pour ice-water in your bed." (A threat executed more than ten times.)

Her insidious campaign spread. The "Please-continue-using-your-fork-to-eat-the-peas, Madeleine" comments (positive reinforcement is a handmaiden to courtesy) were sandwiched between more bouquets thrown to me—"Dear, thanks for grocery shopping," and "thanks for taking out the trash every Thursday."

In a perverse way I felt attacked. Her gratitude disrupted my exercises in self-pity, wherein I suffer in noble silence being the ultimate scullery boy, get no recognition for all the dirty little things I do for others, sacrifice living out my mellow years as a dapper playboy in the south of France, as I was meant to do. (If a woman has the right to charge her mind, a guy has an equal right to feel sorry for himself.)

I was ready to say, "Enough with the politeness" and ask for some help with cooking, setting the table and scrubbing pots and pans when Anastasia and Drusila began breaking from their studying and primping to thank me, too! It was spreading like a cold virus! Finally, my lazy son who hides during Thursday-morning trash-toting time emerged from a closet after the deed was done one day to say, "Dad, thank you for not throwing out the Legos in the front yard." (Had I known they were there, I would have.)

Clearly, an epidemic of politesse was sweeping the household. I noticed even the kids began using terms of endearment on one another—except, of course, when they were at one another's throats, which seldom exceeds 60 percent of their waking hours.

I knew something big was happening when I started hearing comments from outside the family about how polite my children were.

Polite? *My kids?*

At first I took it as a throwaway compliment...you know, something nice to say to fill the ample slack time at PTA meetings. But it kept coming—steady feedback on not just my two daughters, but the Little Lebowski himself started getting raves from moms in his Cub Scout den. One, okay, but three of them?

The evidence was overwhelming. How could I not become a convert? I started prefacing my common cries for help with

Memoirs of a Geezer Dad

"Dearest Molly, would you set the table for me tonight?" She didn't accept my wiles at first, having a keen taste for irony and suspecting me of engaging in what she calls "your usual sarcasm," conveyed to me with narrowed eyes and twisted lips. But in time I became more facile with the sweet nothings and got more help and less static. Moreover, I found my "dears" and "darlings" and "sweets" and (for the boy) "good friend" or "my buddy" had a synergistic effect when combined with the act of "touching," adding a patina of domestic bliss over the reality of domestic mess. Daily life got a lot easier.

I'm proud of my adjustments and pass along the "courtesy trick" with the strongest recommendation. Ultimate credit, though, still accrues to my wife, she of the positive resolve. I must say she is a powerful civilizing presence in our home and has elevated our level of living by showing us how to be kind and thoughtful.

6. Don't Fight Nature

Most little girls like to do little girls things. (Some don't, and that's okay.) Most little boys like to do boys things. (Some don't, and that's okay, too.) I've learned that if it's in them, don't try to take it out of them, because you're wasting your time.

Madeleine was born with a passion for dolls—a natural flowering of maternal instincts that showed themselves in years of collecting. To walk these dolls she acquired a sizeable collection of deceptively flimsy-looking strollers, most of which I met shin-high on nocturnal journeys of bladder relief. (Amazing the abuse these sturdy perambulators can take when vigorously kicked down a hallway.)

Dear things breed more dear things. Soon the dolls were

224

joined by an alarming accumulation of fuzzy, fleecy, cuddly stuffed animals that first covered her bed, then her room, and ultimately overran the house. My attempts to control their numbers by stealthily dropping the occasional stray into a garbage can precipitated such an uproar that I abandoned all efforts at population control. Remarkable how she could miss just one little lamb.

Deliverance came with the arrival of Mimi. Lacking the fauna of her native Labrador to cut her teeth on, the pup took to chewing Madeleine's stuffed animals to bits of cotton and kapok. To put a fine point on it, the dog succeeded where I had failed.

Nature wasn't done with thinning the ranks, though. Puberty came for Madeleine, and the dolls began to disappear, to where she now is down to only an American Girl doll and a Bitty Baby—both collectors' items she assures me. For stuffed animals, she's down to a bear and a cat, both gifts from adults, interestingly.

When I recently asked her where all the cuddlies went, she laconically replied, "I outgrew that, Dad." And so she had…. I just hope that doesn't mean she's given up plans to be a mom.

Girls do become young women soon enough, but boys stay boys for quite a bit longer. I was reminded of this months ago by a matter-of-fact declaration to me by warrior son Franz: "Dad, I like movies with guns and swords in them." As if he had to tell me.

I saw early in his play and television-watching confirmation of the natural linkage between boys, toys and violence. Do boys have an inborn affinity for guns and soldiers and their end purposes? Or does the early exposure to toy weaponry point boys-into-men toward mayhem? Experience tells me each feeds the other.

The three sons of my first marriage were born during the

Memoirs of a Geezer Dad

Vietnam War, and war toys were a flammable social issue in our suburban community. My then-wife and I were somewhat neutral on the subject, but some forward-looking neighbor mothers conspired to ban all war toys from their houses and (perhaps unconsciously) the neighborhood. I doubted that nature could be so easily thwarted. And I got proof when their sons started showing up to play in our house with my boys in what had became a default arsenal of democracy.

Coming completely clean, I confess I actually encouraged my sons' playing of war games. With them I would arrange armies of green plastic soldiers in a backyard Nam jungle of Bermuda grass and then take turns bowling them fatally over with thrown tennis balls or socks. No guilt here whatsoever. I was a boy during World War II when there were good guys and bad guys cleanly defined, and the fate of the world was up for grabs, and evil had to be overthrown by the noblest of us—and the movies showed us violence was the only way. The flicks fired us with patriotism...and, of course, hid war's horrors. While attending to the chore of burning our trash (backyard incinerators were legal and ubiquitous then in Southern California), my buddies and I would collect and put aside all the empty milk cartons we could trash-pick and wait until my mother went shopping. Then out they came—the half-gallon-sized ones transformed into Japanese carriers, the quart-size enemy cruisers, the pint-size escorting destroyers—to become a dread fleet spread out on the green swells of our imagined Philippine Sea. We dive-bombed from above and torpedoed from the side with Ohio blue-tipped matches until the stricken fleet flared and sputtered its last on a choppy green expanse. If Mom still hadn't returned, we turned our wrath to enemies on land. Ten-cent cans of Kwik-lite lit at their plastic tips made excellent flame throwers for dealing with ant colonies dug in on the sands of our backyard Iwo Jima.

226

My Advice to You

Nearly five years in the United States Air Force during the Korean War dampened my martial ardor some, but a certain fascination with weapons stayed with me. On a trip to Spain when my first batch of boys were nine and ten years old, I walked Madrid trying to find presents they would like. And I settled on? Toy Colt .45s and bota bags. "You must be raising a crop of drunken gunfighters," a traveling companion observed. I laughed, but not comfortably.

With my last son Franz, I resolved to stay neutral. I would not encourage him in any martial fantasies, buy him any guns, knives or war toys without his asking—repeatedly—for them. He did, repeatedly. Even as mid-toddler, the sound of TV gunfire would stop him in his tracks for an appreciative stare at the screen. So I caved in. What cannot be denied cannot be withheld. We started with a company of those familiar little green plastic soldiers.

Let nature take its course, I decided. Most men outgrow a participatory interest in warfare, I've noticed, even as their fascination for the subject lingers. I saw the start of that with Franz when he was only five and playing voyeur while I watched History Channel footage of the Normandy invasion.

"I guess those guys in the army don't know they could be skeletons, do they?" Franz asked out of the blue.

Caught off guard, I hesitated before saying, "They do."

"Then why do they go into the army?"

"They had to. Back then we had a draft."

"What's a draft?"

"It's when the government says you have to go into the army and defend your country."

"Will I have to go into the army?"

"No. We don't have the draft anymore. You volunteer for the army now, if you want to...but you don't have to."

He seemed relieved that he was not in immediate peril but

no less perplexed at the prospect that men actually fought wars in which they risked being killed—a conundrum that we have revisited often over the intervening years.

"I think most men who join armies don't think they are going to die," I told him once. He didn't have trouble accepting that. But when I added, "and some probably don't care if they do," he balked.

"That's stupid," he said.

I told him how some men were willing to die (and kill) for an ideal or beliefs they held, but he was not swayed. Why should he be? War with the weapons now available is stupid. It should be unthinkable. That it isn't is prima facie evidence that the whole species, celebrated for its ability to think, isn't thinking. Look around the globe if you have doubts.

My son watched over my shoulder the absorbing and frightening events in Afghanistan and asked me to explain their relevance to him. Clearly, he felt threatened by what he saw and heard from a region of the world armed and in turmoil. I did my parental best to explain the causes of the conflict, even as I found myself downplaying the very real dangers to the whole world posed by terrorists who have answers to all our questions and would gladly give their lives to impose them on us. The boy, who knows all the countries bordering Afghanistan and has taught himself the ethnic composition of the Northern Alliance, listened attentively. But it's plain he's not ready yet to accept the seeming contradiction that war is often necessary to assure peace, and that men who fight wars can be simultaneously horrified and edified by their actions. The bipolar truths of paradox don't register in a nine-year-old's mind.

Perhaps when he's older I can play the literary card and refer him to Stephen Crane and *The Red Badge of Courage* to better explain the ambivalence of men to war. Until then I mean to continue pushing the virtues of skepticism and tolerance at the expense of certitude and rage. Of course, if it turns out we are programmed to kill one another over abstractions, then I rescind my advice. Nature then must be fought, to save the species and my children.

7. Manage Gently Petty Theft

When I was an undergraduate I roomed with two psychology majors who filled my head with strategies they'd picked up on how to take personality and aptitude tests at job-hunting time. All I still retain from those briefings is that, if male, you always tell the shrink or test paper that you took your problems to your father, not your mother. That when asked if you had to be an animal, what would it be, you should answer tigers or race horses (emblematic of the marketplace virtues of aggression and competition), not birds or rabbits who fly and hie away from life's hurly-burly. The third and final "don't" was don't say on the test that you never engaged in petty theft when you were a kid. That question, often sprinkled throughout the test in slightly different wordings, is meant, paradoxically, to validate the test-taker's honesty. The assumption? That everyone stole something when they were young—and those who say they didn't are liars.

Once I accept that even my hyper-honest father must have pinched a penny at least once, I can buy into the dictum. Only my sainted mother dead now for 32 years gets cleared by me of the filching charge. Not that she was perfect. She also happened to be the mother of all kitsch, enamored of corny crockery bowls and statuary and household gewgaws. Her garish collection, which memorably included a hamburger relish set of bowls featuring a puckered pickle face, a weeping onion, and "May O'Naise," has long since been dispersed, probably cheering the depths of a landfill somewhere at this moment. The only surviving piece is a treasured Christmas gift she gave me back in the late 1950s. It's a ceramic dog valet—a cream-colored beagle peppered with black and rust flecks—that holds a wallet in its recessed back, a wristwatch around its upturned nose, one's keys from its upright tail, and, in a little basket between its front paws, my loose change...soon to become someone else's loose change.

For two generations now "Dad's dog" has provided his children with walking-around money. Coins I drop into its recesses stay at a constant level, no matter how much I feed the pup. Every now and then I nab a child in the light-fingered act. And I mildly scold him or her.

You let them off that easily, you're thinking? You've got to crack down on petty crime big time. Make them earn those coins, you're telling me. Put them to work.

Well, I tried that with my first family. Lectured them long on honesty and the virtues of labor. Formulated a plan in which allowances were given for work done. Threatened them with the withdrawal of privileges if it wasn't. I even renamed the posted "Chore Chart" the "Opportunity Chart" to put a positive spin on our quid-pro-quo arrangement.

To little avail. For all the family meetings and follow-up status reports, the work was at best sporadically done, the status of the three accounts always murky, and fights over who was supposed to be doing what sapped much of the family energy. And all the while the ceramic dog's weight-loss problem continued.

Little has changed the second time around. My daughters plead academic demands to get out of work, and because they're pulling As and Bs, I argue from a weakened position. As for the lad, he gets good grades, too, with a minimum of study and a maximum of indolent woolgathering. The dog, meanwhile, holds its lean condition, evidence that the pilfering still goes on.

At a recent birthday celebration, my first generation of sons jocularly recalled past heists in front of me and the second generation. I wanted to object as they passed along tips on tapping Dad's dog without arousing suspicion, how to fish coins out without making a clinking sound that could be heard in an adjacent room, how you should leave a mix of coinage and not pig-out on quarters, how you make deals with one another in advance so the pooch isn't over-milked and always has some silver to show its master. All this said in front of my very ears!

Was I laughing with them? No. I was feeling mighty ambivalent. On the one hand I was pleased that the two sets of offspring separated by different mothers were relating so well to one another. But the seniors teaching the juniors the art of pilferage? What's a geezer father to do?

Live with it. That's the bottom line to my advice on handling petty theft. Sure, employ whatever incentives you can to keep it petty and head-off felonies and the court system. Before making it a federal case, though, try looking the other way. And get yourself a ceramic dog. A small one.

8. About the Hummingbirds and the Bees

"Dad, I saw two hummingbirds, one following the other," Franz, age six and a half, excitedly announced to his father busy at the computer keyboard. "It looked like one, but it was really two stuck together."

"Wow! Imagine that!"

"Why did they do that?"

"I guess because they like each other."

"Were they mating?"

Memoirs of a Geezer Dad

"Probably were."

Long wait. No further questions. Great! Let asexual minds sleep, I say. But what was this about mating? What did he know of that? I would have to put off knowing because I certainly wasn't going on any fishing expedition.

I practice what I preach. Volunteer nothing beyond a narrow honest answer to questions children ask. Needless embellishments become the basis of additional questions and often lead into knowledge they're not ready for. Of course, they'll likely be filled in and led on by those proverbial kids on the street anyway. After which you will doubtless have some correcting to do.

I have found that when the comprehensive showdown does come, it's best to ignore the textbook Latinate diction and go to the gritty language of the street , the no-nonsense Anglo-Saxon lingo. Those are the one-syllable words they've already heard. I just make a point of delivering them in a matter-of-fact, clinical tone of voice, without a lot of editorializing.

It worked famously with my first three sons, who seem now well-adjusted in their relationships. The only editorializing I did was to plug condoms and mention the enhancing value of love when added to mere carnal transactions. No other judgements or advice beyond protecting themselves and their partners. Whatever personal kinks they wanted to add to the enduring mystery were entirely their own business.

And for my second team? Including my daughters? I've proceeded more warily. I'm not so presumptuous as to think I know what's best for them. Or even to know how to begin.

Madeleine flashes the yellow caution light to me regularly. At age six she informed me that she wasn't "into boys...except the one I've got the crush on at school."

"Oh?" was all the tongue-tied geezer could say. Forecast: Woe ahead for me.

Later I found a rudimentary love letter to a boy named Paul, complete with hearts and a portrait (presumably of the boy in question) with an overlarge head.

My stomach churned. Should I confront her? Dig it all out and tell her she was too young to be thinking of boys. I couldn't find the will or the words.

Later that same day she threw acid on my dyspepsia by asking, "Do you know the hardest part of having a new baby?"

Dread froze me. What could this sheltered six-year-old know of labor? "What?" I asked.

"Remembering its name."

Whew! *Quelle* relief!

Temporary.

When Madeleine started walking around the house with a volleyball under her tee shirt, pretending to be pregnant, I recused myself from the sex education of my daughters. Simply not qualified. Turned that weighty responsibility over to their mother. I would confine my tutoring to the Dude, in the basics, and only when called upon. Again, let him add his own wrinkles later, according to his own lights.

9. Flash Them a Flaw or Two

I may patent this one. It's all about breaking that inevitable fall from infallibility every parent goes through. Kids start out by thinking you have all the answers, then gradually find out you don't have more than a clue, that you're just another Joe or Hermione Klutz faking your way through life. It's quite a tumble, believe me!

So why not break the fall by owning up early to a few deficiencies? Cushion the fall by not claiming to know it all. Let them see the chinks in your armor before that time when, as

233

adolescents, they suddenly reduce you in rank from omniscient to incompetent.

I discovered this gambit as a university lecturer—admittedly, too late to do me much good with my first wave of kids. At the lectern, I found it hard to pretend to knowledge I didn't have, as some of my peers did. The sharp students in class always saw through the "my-way, no-further-questions" dogma for what it is—Herr Professor vainly covering up the holes in his scholar's gown. Better, I found, to admit to the lack of an answer and then invite the students to join you on a Socratic chase of the truth. They really appreciated the chance to join the hunt and show you they just might know something you didn't. And they often did and do.

I applied the method to my second family with instant success. I let them know when they were toddlers that I couldn't draw. I can't. Not a straight line, not an imperfect circle. Nothing. Never could. I spent my early years secretly hiding the fact from everyone (except my grammar school teachers who gave me a gift C in art), just as I have buried the failings of not knowing how to whistle or snap my fingers. I confessed my fine art limitations to my second brood early on, and they loved it! Being better at something than Dad! And bless their charitable hearts, they wanted to teach the old man how to draw—starting with a cat. No matter how hard I still try, my cats always come out looking like pancaked hyenas—a source of much family mirth every time I flunk the course.

More valuable, however, is what my children teach me of the brave new electronic world that engulfs and often confounds seniors my age, who first saw the cutting edge of technology with indoor plumbing and the Curtiss P-40. Our ultimate comfort zone remains sitting in front of the Philco listening to *Lum and Abner*.

Personally, I like to think I'm half-wired. At least I know a

CD from a space-directed missile and that a DVD is not a social disease. Moreover, I'm semi-facile with my iMac, go online regularly for research data and to do my banking, word-process almost daily. Just put me in the company of unplugged geezers and geezerettes and watch me swagger! Words like "modem" and "scanner" and "spam" pepper my speech as I nag them to get with the modern program—"it saves so much time once you get the hang of it."

But see me back in the company of my children, and you might mistake me for a chip-age orphan in need of care. They have to program the VCR for me. Get the satellite signal back. And when I can't access a file or the printer goes on the blink, my desperate mayday call brings them running with knowledge they seem to have absorbed through their young pores and— often as not—with a solution to my problem.

I always make a point of thanking them volubly, out of genuine appreciation for their help and also so I can watch them puff up with pride and, if I'm not mistaken, affection. They love mentoring me. As I do them. It's life on Win-Win Street, and it runs two ways.

10. Keep the Back Door Open

When I was a child, I had trouble with the prodigal son parable. Why should the debauched guy get the royal welcome and fattened calf for coming home broke when the dutiful son had stayed home, worked hard and got nothing extra for his pains. Didn't seem fair.

Now I am old and I understand. Retrieving what is lost is just as great a cause for celebration as keeping what is secure.

I won't list here the many clashes I've had with my three older sons when I was tempted to give up on them. I'm just thankful that in our hottest moments we always left open the back door to reconciliation…a "back channel" as they put it in diplomatic circles, where tenuous contact is maintained, through a third party if necessary.

While I still favor a magic pill that would put fourteen-year-olds to sleep until they turned 19, when they would awake mature and none the worse for their slumber, I cringe when I hear parents say they are disowning a child. Or want no further contact with a son or daughter. No doubt some children earn their exile…or maybe the parent is an unfit role model. Just don't burn the bridge is my advice. Whether we like it or not, change rules the universe. We change, as do those we love or have loved. And sometimes change brings back what's been lost. And that is love.

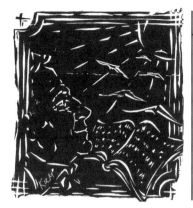

Chapter 19

Concluding Unscientific Postscript

FRANCIS BACON GOT it right when he wrote, "He that hath wife and children hath given hostages to fortune." Though I've always suspected he was motivated more by his own march to a deviant drummer than by any desire to advise wavering bachelors, the caveat to would-be parents still stands.

Over recent years a few friends have asked whether I would recommend geezer fatherhood to others. The quick answer—no. If you survived the first round intact, you've earned the right to pursue your hedonistic ways through your waning days unemcumbered. If you never had a child and waited until achieving senior-citizen status to entertain the option, don't even consider it. Parenting is a young man's profession; old guys simply aren't tough enough.

One friend mustered the nerve to ask whether I personally regretted having a second family at my age. My answer, more slowly arrived at, was another "no"—a firm no. The more I thought about it, the more I realized I was destined to become a geezer father.

To say why takes some digging through the strata of my mind. Up top are those negative reasons that belong under the banner "What Better Things Did I Have To Do?" They make a great antidote to the fallacy of the presumed better road not taken.

I'm of the wrong political persuasion to spend my golden years complaining about high taxes at the shuffleboard court.

Memoirs of a Geezer Dad

Sunning myself among the sand-scattered bikinis of the Cote D'Azur would be a classic case of being in the right place at the wrong time. Slowing down and blimping up luxury cruising the world (already done, courtesy Uncle Sam and a stint as a free-loading travel writer) would only exacerbate existing health problems.

Digging deeper, I realize that I'm restless still, fearing death and abhorring loneliness even after turning 70. I once thought we all grew into wisdom as we aged…and conquered our fears. Instead, I find myself among the many who persist in their innate eccentricities and are made grotesques by them. So be it. At some unconscious level I probably chose a second family so I would not live alone and die alone, unloved and unattended.

There are other less-than-obvious benefits. This geezer father is too busy and harried to slip into the usual depressive mood so common to certain idle seniors packing around Northern European genes. You especially don't have to worry about Empty Nest Depression; one flock out and another one in—and chances are you'll check out before they fly off. Moreover, you may not require nursing care insurance; presuming your own can put up with your last sordid needs. Taking the rosy view a bit further, you even find you can tolerate little-boy noises—all those whoops, bellows, squawks, strangled belches and failed-fart sounds, not to mention those that can't be ascribed to living things or the inanimate world. So in love with the senses am I.

That admission behind me, I confess to skipping over one major downside to geezer parenthood that I must acknowledge here at book's end. It is the lack—and the loss therefrom—of grandparents for my young hostages. I first became truly sensitive to that loss when I became a grandparent myself six years ago with the birth of a handsome grandson, Dane, courtesy of

238

Concluding Unscientific Postscript

my son Karl and his wife Aliki; three years later they added to the grandparent treasury a winsome little red-headed girl, Makana. Such a lucky pair to have—thanks to today's longer lifespans—four doting grandparents to lavish love and extend those extra helping hands and watchful eyes.

Not so blessed my second generation of kids. My mother and father died years before Molly and Madeleine and Franz even became possibilities. Their maternal grandfather died when Franz was a baby, and their surviving grandmother is chronically ill and reclusive. That void, I've found, leads to confusion and embarrassment on "Grandparent's Day"—a popular institution in grammar school these days. The greater loss, though, is their being denied the company of your own mother and father after they have mellowed into that natural harmony between generations one removed…grandma and grandpa finding tolerance and a purpose in spoiling grandchildren who carry their hopes and genes and sometimes their names into the future.

The loss is double-edged. You also regret that your own mother and father cannot see what has come after them, heirs in part of their wit or looks or quirks or virtues. (Vices are generally overlooked in such comparisons.) I wish my mother could have seen her prized red hair (absent in four children and her first ten grandchildren) pop up in my first daughter Molly, who is otherwise a close facsimile of her in freckled Celtic complexion; my mother would appreciate her old-fashioned, lady-like ways as belonging to a gentler time. In Madeleine she would see the same red hair in a shy and determined lass who bears her first name as her second, Jeannette; she would especially relate to her granddaughter's love of infants and animals. And I regret that my father cannot see the super-athlete I never was for him in the long-boned lankiness of Franz, who swings a mean baseball bat and pulls down basketball rebounds with consummate grace. Never to be, even as fleeting memories taken to the grave.

To assure that I will be remembered, I'm building a small domestic monument in my study, just to the left of my iMac. My son Karl, who owns Gentle Giant Studios in Burbank, California, broke from his bronzing of the celebrity likes of George Lucas and Hugh Heffner to make a bust of his father for my sixty-ninth birthday. It will be focal to the shrine, surrounded by the books and verse I've written, a portrait of me at age 35, slim and in my prime, my degrees framed in non-reflective glass on the wall, alongside my Honorable Discharge, my Phi Beta Kappa key, and my Whittier Union High School varsity letter W in baseball. Very convenient to my family, who may visit the shrine at any time, burn votive candles if they wish, communicate with me if they can. I have promised to respond from the other side if allowed more than that one phone call to my attorney.

Initially, I had hoped to grace the bust with a pithy epigram that summed up my life's thinking about being and meaning…only to find Shakespeare—no surprise—has already framed it in an eloquent sentence: "We are such stuff as dreams are made on, and our little life is rounded with a sleep."

No improving on that.

And the disposition of the remains? My heirs can van the carcass off to the Santa Anita Racetrack Infield where I believe I have purchased by now a plot beneath the pansies under the Parimutuel Layaway Plan.

I close this memoir expressing a pair of deep regrets. One is that ending it means my own life is winding down, and I probably will not be around long to help my survivors through the hard times sure to come; the other is that it took me so long to accept what the poets long have told us—that only the prospect of death gives life meaning and validates art.

Concluding Unscientific Postscript

Was geezer fatherdom worth it after all? After the decisions and revisions and all the other Prufrockian second thoughts? Absolutely. How could I have lived without the daily company of my six wonderful children, three sired in the 1960s and the other three in my late middle age and after? When I leave them, they will have my beloved wife to pick up my love for them all and apply it to those born and yet to be born into the line. *Amor omnia vincit.* In the end, there is only love, active and remembered, to warm the chill of a cooling universe.

Book Design by Paulette Boudreau
Illustrations by Eric, Kurt, Karl, Kelly, Molly,
Madeleine, Franz and Larry L. Meyer;
Timarie Lawrence; and Paulette Boudreau

The Text Is
11.5/14 Goudy Old Style

Printed on acid-free paper in the
United States of America

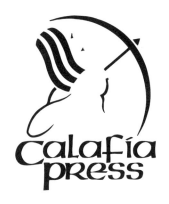

Huntington Beach, California
calafiapress.com

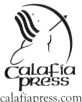

Calafia press

calafiapress.com

Quick Order Form

POSTAL ORDERS:	Calafia Press PO Box 5610 Huntington Beach, CA 92615-5610
FAX ORDERS:	(714) 964-1554 Send this form.
TELEPHONE ORDERS:	(714) 964-0212

Please send me _____copy (copies) of
No Paltry Thing: Memoirs of a Geezer Dad
at $22.00 per copy. I enclosed a check or money
order in the amount of $_____.

SEND TO:

Name _____

Address _____

City _____

State _____ ZIP _____

Sales tax: Please add 7.75% for books shipped to California addresses.

Shipping by air: U.S.: $4.00 for first book; $2.00 for each additional.